NOVEL INSIGHTS ON CHRONIC KIDNEY DISEASE, ACUTE KIDNEY INJURY AND POLYCYSTIC KIDNEY DISEASE

Edited by **Soundarapandian Vijayakumar**

Novel Insights on Chronic Kidney Disease, Acute Kidney Injury and Polycystic Kidney Disease
Edited by Soundarapandian Vijayakumar

Published by InTech
Janeza Trdine 9, 51000 Rijeka, Croatia

Publishing Process Manager Petra Nenadic

Technical Editor Teodora Smiljanic

Cover Designer InTech Design Team

Additional hard copies can be obtained from orders@intechopen.com

Novel Insights on Chronic Kidney Disease, Acute Kidney Injury and Polycystic Kidney Disease, Edited by Soundarapandian Vijayakumar
p. cm.
ISBN 978-953-51-0234-2

For EU product safety concerns:
IN TECH d.o.o., Prolaz Marije Krucifikse Kozulić 3, 51000 Rijeka, Croatia,
info@intechopen.com or visit our website at intechopen.com.

Meet the editor

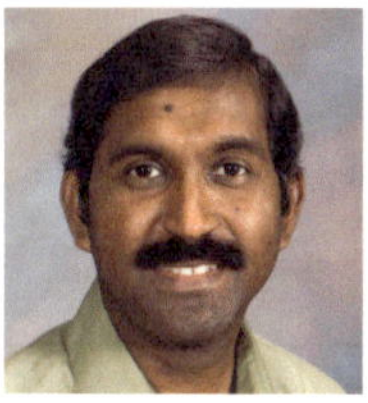

Dr. Vijayakumar is currently an Assistant Professor in the Departments of Pediatrics and Pharmacology & Physiology at the University of Rochester. He has held research positions at the Columbia University in the City of New York as well as the University of Texas Southwestern Medical Center, Dallas, TX. As a young scientist, he has spent time at the University of Ulm, Germany and International Center for Theoretical Physics, Italy. He has published in several leading journals such as the Journal of Cell Biology and Journal of Clinical Investigation, primarily on the role of hensin in acid-base physiology. His research has mainly focused on the cell biology and physiology of kidney collecting duct and his current work is on the extracellular matrix abnormalities in polycystic kidney disease.

Contents

Preface

Chronic kidney disease (CKD) has been recently recognized by the United Nations as a major non-communicable disease that poses significant health burden to the world population. This book offers novel insights on topics such as congenital obstructive nephropathy, cerebral-renal salt wasting, and the role of hemoglobin variability in clinical outcomes of CKD which are not very often discussed in the literature. Two related topics, primary aldosteronism and the role of renin-angiotensin-aldosterone system in the development of hypertension in CKD patients are also discussed. Acute Kidney Injury (AKI), characterized by a rapid reduction in kidney function, is more common in hospitalized patients and is an independent risk factor for mortality. Dr. Khanal Namrata discusses the epidemiology, causes and outcome of obstetric acute kidney injury in this book. Polycystic Kidney Diseases (PKD) are a group of genetic diseases affecting nearly 12 million people worldwide and there has been a significant interest and progress in the understanding of these diseases. Two often overlooked topics, the role of extracellular matrix abnormalities in PKD cystogenesis and progression, and the role of angiogenesis in ADPKD pathogenesis provide critical insights into these topics. With comprehensive and insightful reviews by eminent clinicians and scientists in the field, this book is a valuable tool for nephrologists.

Dr. S. Vijayakumar, Ph.D
Pediatric Nephrology
University of Rochester Medical Center
USA

Part 1

Acute and Chronic Kidney Diseases

1

Congenital Obstructive Nephropathy: Clinical Perspectives and Animal Models

Susan E. Ingraham and Kirk M. McHugh
Department of Pediatrics, Division of Pediatric Nephrology, The Ohio State University and The Research Institute at Nationwide Children's Hospital, Columbus, Ohio, USA

1. Introduction

Congenital obstructive nephropathy is the leading cause of pediatric chronic kidney disease (CKD). Consequently, it engenders a tremendous societal burden in terms of morbidity and mortality and in health care expenses over the lifespan of affected patients. The challenges clinicians face in the diagnosis, prognosis, and treatment of congenital obstructive nephropathy illustrate the utility of developing effective experimental models for the study of this complex disease process. In this review, we characterize congenital obstructive nephropathy with its myriad causes and manifestations, outline current standards of diagnosis and care, and discuss experimental animal models with relevance in unraveling clinical conundrums and molecular mechanisms of this important renal disease.

Congenital obstructive nephropathy is a complex process of pathologic changes in kidney development and function that arise when antegrade urine flow is impaired beginning *in utero*. The term *congenital obstructive uropathy* is frequently used to describe this condition. However, every urologic obstruction - whether anatomic, mechanical, or functional - should be approached with the knowledge that obstruction can affect the kidneys. For this reason, we prefer the term *congenital obstructive nephropathy*.

Intrinsic anatomic obstructions may occur in isolation or accompanied by other pathology such as renal hypodysplasia. Functional obstructions also occur, which may be transient and self-resolving, or chronic with potentially profound consequences on renal function. Although the etiologies of congenital obstructive nephropathy are myriad, any restriction of urine flow has the potential to produce hydronephrosis, altered renal development, and progression of CKD. This direct link between obstructed urine flow and abnormal kidneys represents a central paradigm of urogenital pathogenesis that has far-reaching implications (Woolf & Thiruchelvam, 2001).

2. Epidemiology of congenital obstructive nephropathy

Congenital obstructive nephropathy is the most common cause of CKD in children and is among the top three etiologies of pediatric end-stage renal disease (ESRD; NAPRTCS, 2009).

Congenital obstructive nephropathy is often grouped with renal agenesis, hypoplasia/dysplasia and other abnormalities as a heterogeneous entity termed *congenital anomalies of the kidney and urinary tract* (CAKUT). CAKUT is relatively common, affecting up to 2% of pregnancies (Ismaili et al., 2003; Wiesel et al., 2005). CAKUT accounts for 51% of childhood CKD in North America (NAPRTCS, 2009), and similar frequencies in registry data from around the world (Neild, 2009a). Among the diagnoses within the broad category of CAKUT, obstructive disease carries the greatest risk for developing ESRD (Sanna-Cherchi et al., 2009). The association of renal hypodysplasia and impaired glomerular filtration rate with urological obstruction is well-established. More subtle renal changes such as hypertension, impaired sodium/water handling, and acidosis are also common (Farnham et al., 2005; Gillenwater et al., 1975). Thus the full clinical impact of congenital obstructive nephropathy is immense.

3. Classification of congenital obstructive nephropathy

The timing, extent, etiology, and location of impaired urine flow are important considerations in describing and classifying the causes of obstructive nephropathy. One of the most important and useful distinctions is the anatomic level at which the obstruction occurs - namely, the upper urinary tract (kidney or ureter) versus the lower urinary tract (bladder, bladder outlet or urethra). Upper urinary tract lesions have little potential to affect the contralateral kidney, whereas lower tract anomalies generally put both kidneys at risk.

3.1 Upper urinary tract obstructions

Congenital obstructions of the upper urinary tract include ureteropelvic junction (UPJ) and ureterovesical junction (UVJ) obstructions, as well as obstructing ureteroceles and other anomalies of ureteric structure or position.

3.1.1 Ureteropelvic junction obstruction

UPJ obstruction is the most common congenital urological obstruction (Figure 1). It occurs in one of every 1000-2000 births, with a 3:1 male predominance. Obstruction is bilateral in 20-25% of cases (Woodward & Frank, 2002). Congenital UPJ obstructions usually arise from an adynamic proximal ureteral segment. This dysfunctional segment of the ureter often exhibits abnormal distribution of collagen and/or smooth muscle, and may show altered innervation or vasculature (Hosgor et al., 2005; Payabvash et al., 2007; Yoon et al., 1998). Less common intrinsic causes of UPJ obstruction include a convoluted ureteral course and deformations of the mucosa, including valve-like folds or polyps. UPJ obstruction may also arise from extrinsic compression of the proximal ureter by another structure such as aberrant vasculature or fibrous bands.

3.1.2 Ureterovesical junction obstruction

UVJ obstruction, or primary obstructive megaureter, arises when urine flow is restricted at or near the insertion of the ureter into the bladder (Figure 2). This is the second most common site of congenital obstruction, after the UPJ (Brown et al., 1987; Reinberg et al.,

1991). UVJ obstruction is four times more common in males and arises more often on the left, with bilateral obstructions occurring in up to 25% of cases (Gimpel et al., 2010; Woodward & Frank, 2002). Like UPJ obstruction, UVJ obstruction is typically associated with an adynamic ureteric segment that fails to propagate effective urine flow.

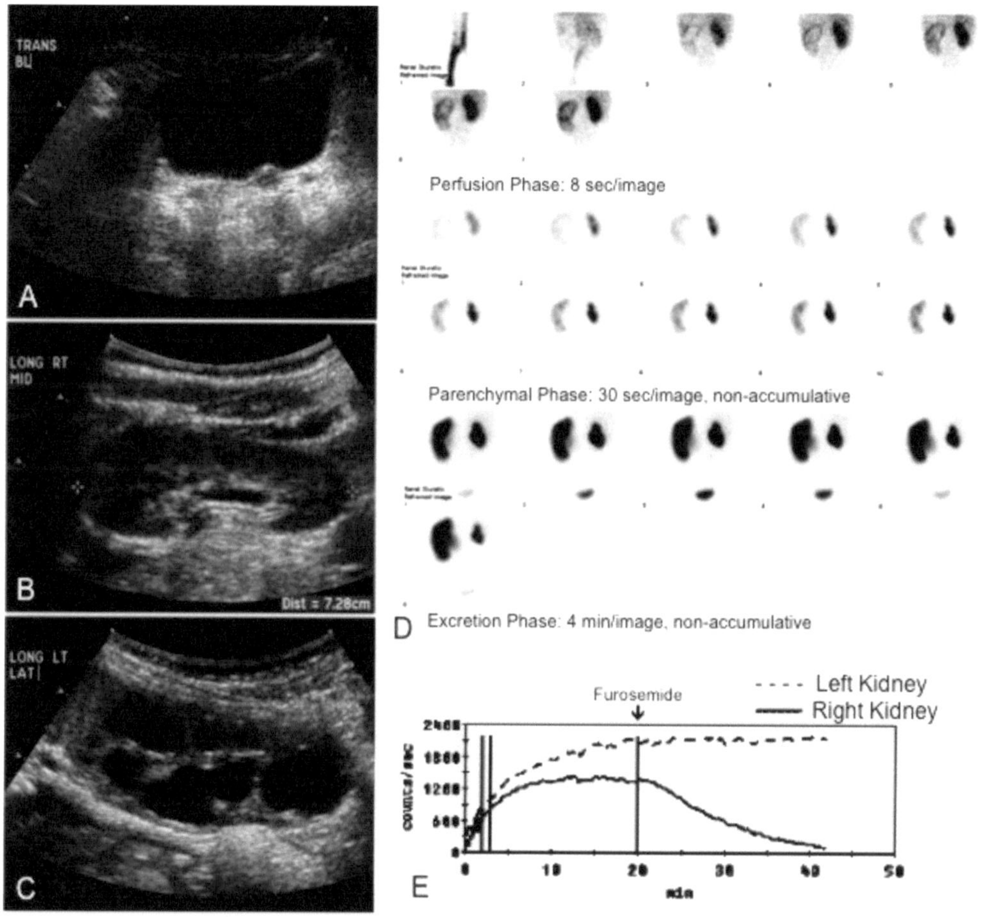

Fig. 1. Radiological findings associated with UPJ obstruction in an 18 month old female. Left hydronephrosis was detected prenatally, and the patient had normal postnatal renal function with no vesicoureteral reflux (VUR). She was managed conservatively, with gradual improvement in hydronephrosis on serial imaging studies through age 15 months. However, at 18 months of age hydronephrosis worsened. **A - C.** Ultrasound of urinary bladder (A), right (B) and left (C) kidneys. The bladder (A) is normal in conformation with normal wall thickness, and no hydroureter is seen. The right kidney (B) is structurally normal with slight pelviectasis. The left kidney (C) demonstrates marked hydronephrosis with blunted calyces and thinned parenchyma, which had worsened from previous findings of moderate but improving hydronephrosis. **D and E.** Technetium-99m MAG3 diuretic renal scan using the F+20 protocol confirmed a left ureteropelvic junction obstruction. Sequential posterior images of the abdomen and pelvis (D) are grouped into perfusion, parenchymal, and excretion phases. Ten milligrams of furosemide were administered 20 minutes after tracer injection. With injection of the tracer, there is bolus visualization of the inferior vena

cava, followed by prompt visualization of renal parenchyma bilaterally. On the right side, there is prompt cortical transit and accumulation in a normal-caliber collecting system followed by appropriate washout. Renogram curve (E) shows a normal right drainage half-time ($T_{1/2}$) of 8.9 minutes. On the left side, the kidney is enlarged with central photopenia consistent with hydronephrosis. Cortical transit is slightly delayed on the left compared to the right. In the excretion phase, tracer accumulates in the hydronephrotic collecting system but there is no washout of the radiopharmaceutical from the left kidney. Left $T_{1/2}$ was not reached in the duration of the study. The patient subsequently underwent left pyeloplasty for UPJ obstruction.

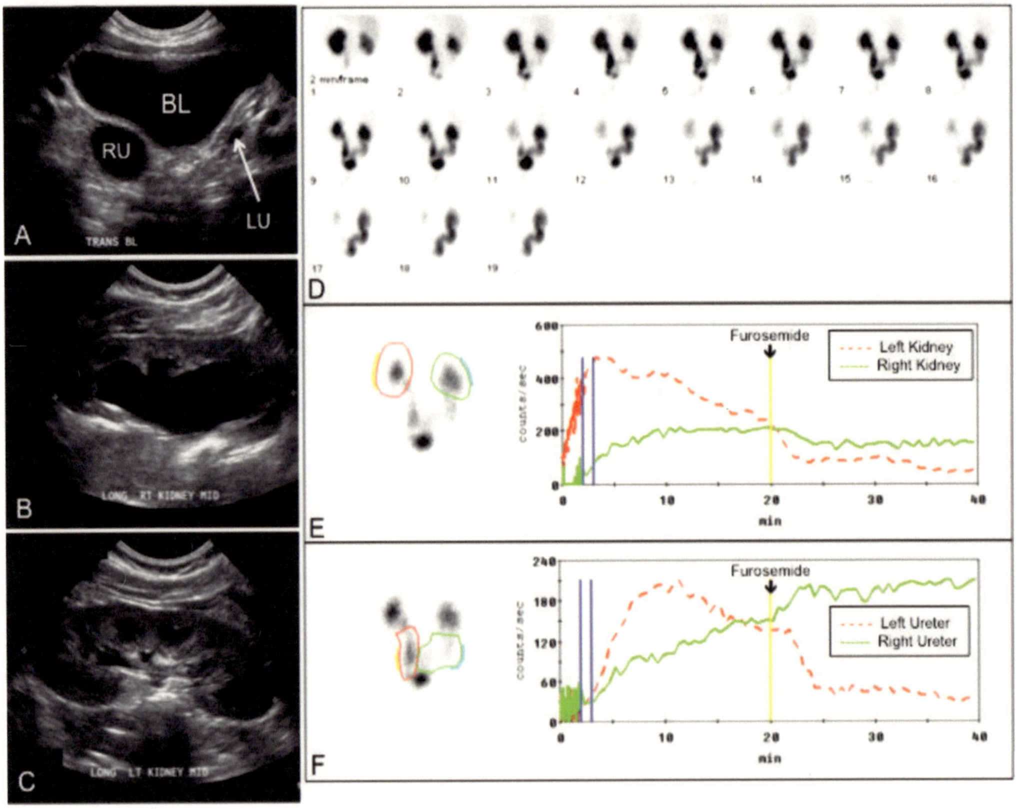

Fig. 2. Radiological findings associated with UVJ obstruction in a 4 month old male. **A - C.** Ultrasound of urinary bladder (A), right (B) and left (C) kidneys. The bladder (BL) is normal in conformation with a smooth wall of normal thickness. Bilateral distal hydroureter is seen, greater on the right (RU) than the left (LU). The right kidney (B) is moderately hydronephrotic with well-preserved parenchyma. The left kidney (C) demonstrates normal echotexture and no hydronephrosis, but urothelial thickening is seen. **D - F.** Technetium-99m MAG3 diuretic renal scan using the F+20 protocol confirmed a right UVJ obstruction. Sequential posterior images are shown for the excretion phase only (D). Renogram curves are illustrated for both kidneys (E) as well as for both ureters (F). Appropriate excretion is observed in the left kidney and ureter both before and after administration of furosemide. On the right side, minimal excretion is demonstrated prior to and following the diuretic. Renal $T_{1/2}$ is 2.3 minutes on the left and never reached on the right.

3.1.3 Ureterocele

Ureteroceles are cystic dilations of the submucosal or intravesical segment of a ureter (Figure 3). If the opening to the ureterocele is stenotic or ectopically positioned, obstruction often results. The prevalence of ureterocele is 1 in 5000 newborns. Unlike the majority of obstructive lesions, ureteroceles demonstrate a female predominance (Woodward & Frank, 2002). Ureteroceles are often associated with a duplex collecting system and/or ectopic ureteral insertion. Depending on the location, configuration and size, unilateral ureteroceles may cause bilateral obstruction. Bilateral ureteroceles are present in 20-50% of cases (Pohl et al., 2007).

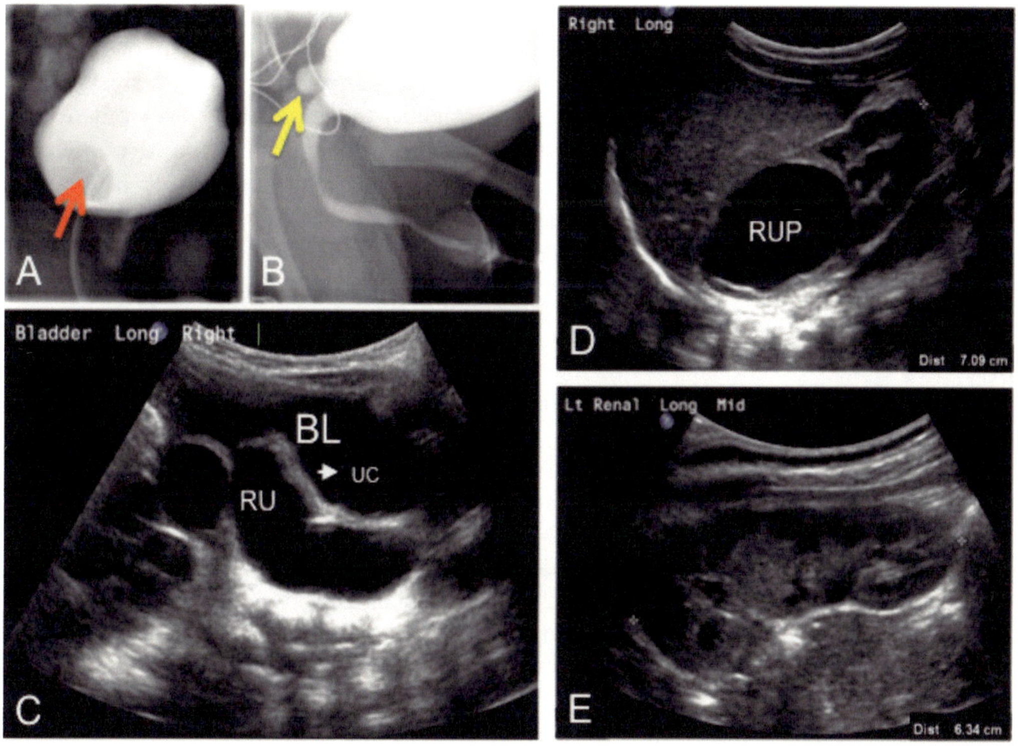

Fig. 3. Radiological findings associated with ureterocele in a 6 day old male. **A and B.** Voiding cystourethrogram (VCUG). Filling image (A) shows the ureterocele as an ovoid filling defect (red arrow). Voiding image (B) shows eversion of the ureterocele (yellow arrow) through an ectopic ureteral insertion, resembling a congenital paraurethral diverticulum. **C – E.** Ultrasound of urinary bladder (C), right (D) and left (E) kidneys. The bladder (BL, image C) is minimally distended but demonstrates smooth walls of normal thickness. Within the bladder, the thin rounded septation (white arrowhead) delineating the ureterocele (UC) is seen. A markedly dilated right distal ureter (RU) is also evident on this lateral, longitudinal view. The right hydroureter is associated with right upper pole hydronephrosis (RUP, image D) in a duplex right kidney. There is minimal hydronephrosis in the right lower pole duplex moiety. A duplex kidney is also observed on the left (E), with no hydronephrosis.

3.1.4 Other upper urinary tract obstructions

Although less common than UPJ or UVJ obstructions, congenital obstructions can arise elsewhere within the kidney or along the course of the ureter. Examples include infundibular or infundibulopelvic stenosis, which may be idiopathic or associated with Beckwith-Wiedemann or Bardet-Biedl syndrome; anomalous ureteric position, such as a retroiliac or retrocaval course; and mid-ureteral stricture.

3.2 Lower urinary tract obstructions

There are several congenital anomalies that result in chronic lower urinary tract obstruction, the most familiar being posterior urethral valves (PUV). Other inborn causes of lower urinary tract obstruction include urethral atresia, stenosis or hypoplasia; anterior urethral valves; urethral diverticula; and cloacal anomalies. Congenital lower urinary tract obstructions put both kidneys at risk for abnormalities in fetal renal development and impaired renal function, and may be associated with oligohydramnios and pulmonary hypoplasia. Congenital lower urinary tract obstructions may also result in bladder dysfunction, ultimately leading to a secondary functional obstruction that may require careful management to optimize renal outcomes.

3.2.1 Posterior urethral valves

PUV, also known as *congenital obstructing posterior urethral membrane,* is found in 1 out of 5000-8000 live births, and occurs only in males (King, 1985). Oligohydramnios is a common consequence, and renal dysplasia may also be present. Using postnatal fluoroscopic VCUG, the gold standard for diagnosis of PUV and other lower urinary tract obstructions (Riedmiller et al., 2001), the classic finding for PUV is a linear filling defect in the column of radiocontrast filling a markedly dilated posterior urethra. However, this distinct linear radiolucent band corresponding to the "valve" is not always seen, because the obstructing membrane can become distended and take on a more sail-like or windsock appearance, as shown in Figure 4. Secondary VUR is found in 25-50% of PUV cases (Agarwal, 1999). In a subset of patients, unilateral VUR may provide a "pop-off" effect, whereby renal tissue and function on the non-refluxing side is preserved at the expense of severe dysplasia and dysfunction in the refluxing kidney (Greenfield et al., 1983).

3.2.2 Urethral atresia, stenosis, or hypoplasia

Although PUV is the most common cause of congenital lower urinary tract obstruction postnatally, detailed postmortem analysis of fetuses with megacystis and hyperechogenic kidneys showed that isolated severe lower urinary tract obstruction before 25 weeks' gestation was as likely to be due to urethral atresia or stenosis as PUV (Robyr et al., 2005). Urethral atresia may arise in association with complex collections of other genitourinary and/or gastrointestinal anomalies. Moreover, urethral atresia may be a cause of bladder outlet obstruction in females whereas PUV is not. Urethral atresia is incompatible with life unless an alternative connection between the bladder and the amniotic sac is present. Prenatal surgical decompression has been performed to relieve this obstruction, although a spontaneous fistula or patent urachus may also provide the necessary bladder drainage

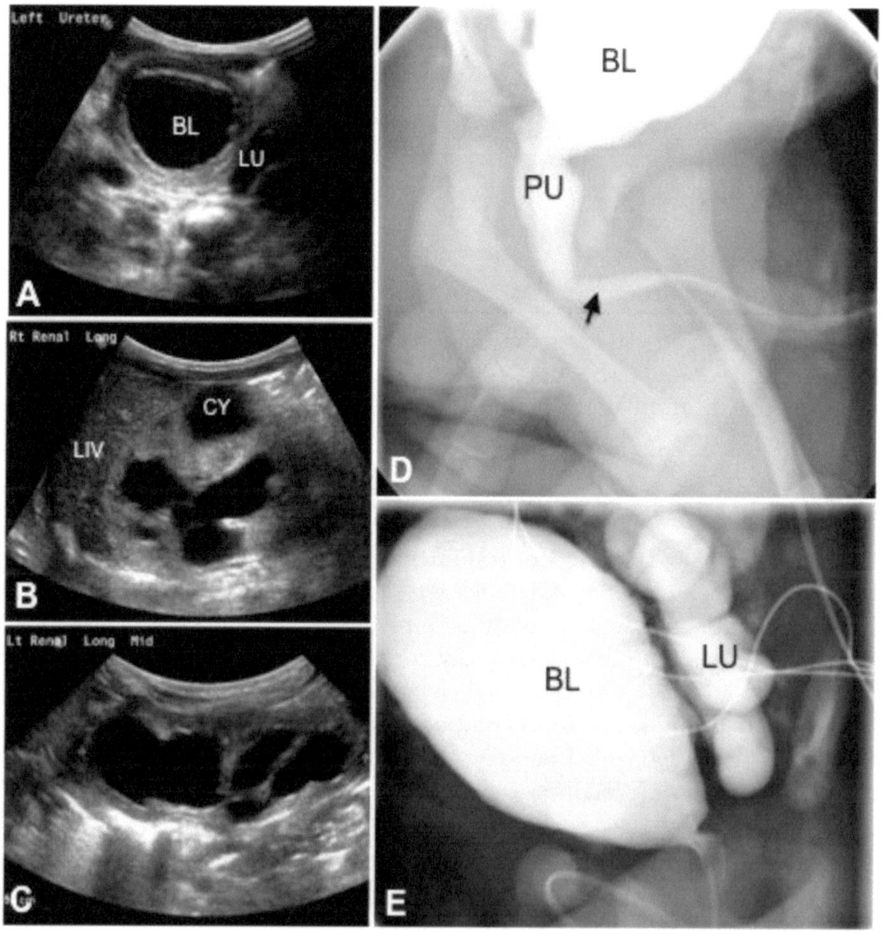

Fig. 4. Radiological findings associated with PUV in a 2 day old male. **A - C.** Ultrasound of urinary bladder (A), right (B) and left (C) kidneys. The bladder (BL) is rounded with a thickened and trabeculated wall. This patient had severe hydroureter bilaterally, although only the left ureter (LU) is clearly observed in image A. Moderate to severe hydronephrosis is present bilaterally, with thinning of the cortex, increased echogenicity relative to the liver (LIV), and poor corticomedullary differentiation. One fluid-filled area (CY) in the right kidney did not clearly communicate with the collecting system, and likely represents a large cyst. **D and E.** VCUG. The lobulated and undulating contours of the urinary bladder (BL) reflect thickening and trabeculation of the bladder wall. The posterior urethra (PU) is dilated. Rather than the classic abrupt transition to a normal caliber anterior urethra, this patient has the "wind-sock" appearance generated by distal prolapse or distention of the valve membrane (arrow). VUR into a tortuous and dilated left ureter (LU) is obvious.

(Gonzalez et al., 2001; Herndon & Casale, 2002). An association between urethral atresia and prune belly syndrome has been recognized (Reinberg et al., 1993). Progression to ESRD is common, although not universal, in surviving patients with urethral atresia (Gonzalez, et al., 2001).

3.2.3 Prolapsing ureterocele

Large ureteroceles can prolapse through the urethra, which may result in bladder outlet obstruction. This is most frequently an acquired condition, although rarely prolapse may occur *in utero*, leading to features of congenital obstructive nephropathy (Sozubir et al., 2003).

3.2.4 Other urethral obstructions

Urethral diverticula and anterior urethral valves are rare causes of infravesicular obstruction. Interestingly, although bladder pathology and variable degrees of hydroureteronephrosis result, renal function is usually not impaired after surgical correction of the obstruction (Arena et al., 2009; Gupta & Srinivas, 2000; Rawat et al., 2009).

3.3 Functional obstruction

Functional urological obstructions are conditions that result in impaired antegrade urine flow without evidence of a physical blockage. In many patients, the situation may be transient and can ultimately resolve without intervention, in which case a specific etiology may never be identified. In other cases a functional obstruction may result from myogenic or neurogenic causes, which can result in lifelong voiding dysfunction as well as significant renal impairment. Examples include conditions such as congenital neurogenic bladder (Ewalt & Bauer, 1996), congenital non-neurogenic neurogenic bladder (Vidal et al., 2009), and prune belly syndrome (Woodhouse et al., 1982).

3.4 Multisystem conditions associated with obstruction or voiding dysfunction

3.4.1 Prune belly syndrome

Prune belly syndrome (Figure 5), also known as Eagle-Barrett syndrome, consists of the triad of underdeveloped abdominal wall musculature, urinary tract dilatation, and undescended testicles (Eagle & Barrett, 1950). Postnatally, urinary obstruction in prune belly syndrome is often functional rather than anatomic in nature. Prune belly syndrome has an incidence of 3.8 per 100,000 male births (Routh et al., 2010). The condition also occurs rarely in females, albeit necessarily lacking cryptorchidism (Reinberg, et al., 1991). Secondary VUR is present in 85% of patients with prune belly syndrome, and associated anomalies of the gastrointestinal, pulmonary, skeletal, and/or cardiac systems are common (Strand, 2004).

Two major theories, which are not mutually exclusive, have been advocated regarding the development of prune belly syndrome. One proposes that the condition arises from a fundamental flaw in mesoderm development (Straub & Spranger, 1981), while the other suggests that prune belly syndrome originates from a severe fetal urethral obstruction that results in massive distention of the bladder, degeneration of the abdominal wall musculature, and interruption of testicular descent (Pagon et al., 1979).

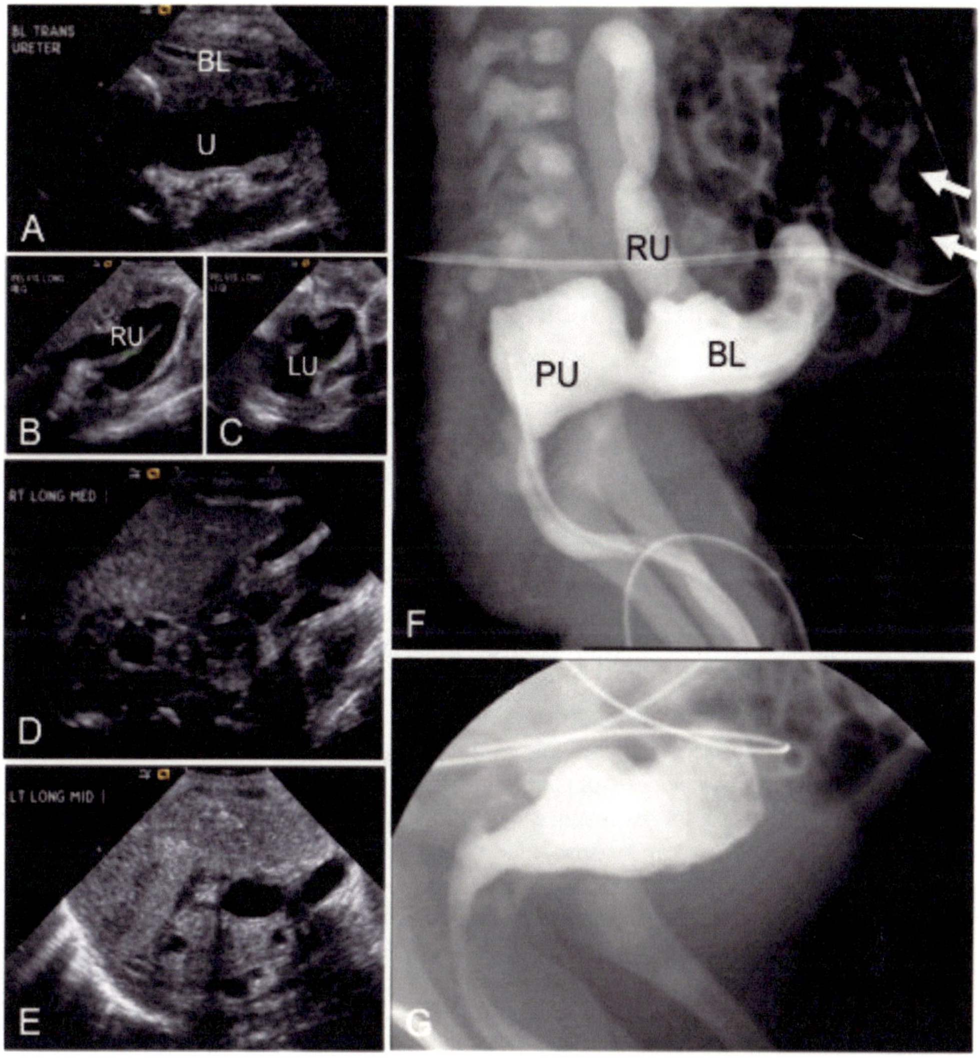

Fig. 5. Radiological findings associated with prune belly syndrome in a 2 day old male. **A - E.** Ultrasound of urinary bladder (A), right (B) and left (C) ureters, right (D) and left (E) kidneys. The bladder (BL) is decompressed but bladder wall thickness is normal. Tortuous dilated ureters (U, RU, LU) are observed bilaterally in the lower abdomen. The kidneys are dysplastic and amorphous in appearance, with cysts of varying sizes. There is no corticomedullary differentiation in either kidney. **F.** VCUG. The protuberant abdomen resulting from lack of abdominal wall musculature is evident from the position of bowel loops (arrows) on this lateral view. This patient has an unusual configuration of the bladder, bladder base and posterior urethra. There is absence of the normal prostate and a very distended posterior urethra (PU) connecting to a dysplastic-appearing bladder (BL). No evidence of true PUV was found on this or any subsequent investigations. Reflux is observed into the distended right ureter (RU) but not the left. **G.** VCUG from another patient 10 days postnatally shows a more typical trabeculated bladder with the characteristic tubular shape of the bladder base in prune belly syndrome.

3.4.2 Spina bifida

Approximately 50% of children with myelomeningocele have detrusor-bladder sphincter dyssynergy, resulting in a functional bladder outlet obstruction and development of hydronephrosis (Anderson & Travers, 1993). These patients can develop the same complications as those with anatomical obstructions, including upper urinary tract dilatation, VUR, incomplete bladder emptying, recurrent urinary tract infections, and CKD (van Gool et al., 2001).

4. Diagnosis of congenital obstructive nephropathy

4.1 Prenatal ultrasound

In developed countries, antenatal diagnosis of congenital urinary obstructions is often made in mid-gestation (at 18-20 weeks), when many pregnant women undergo a detailed prenatal ultrasound. Megacystis with or without oligohydramnios is the characteristic ultrasound finding of lower urinary tract obstruction, whereas hydronephrosis may signal upper or lower urinary tract obstruction. Hydronephrosis is the most commonly detected anomaly on prenatal ultrasound, found in as many as 4.5% of fetuses (Ismaili, et al., 2003). Prenatal hydronephrosis may result from non-obstructive processes such as primary VUR or physiologic dilatation as well as from obstruction. Differentiating obstruction from non-obstructive causes of congenital hydronephrosis is critical because the prognosis and management vary significantly among these conditions. Factors for consideration in assessing fetal hydronephrosis include gestational age; gender; whether the finding is unilateral or bilateral; the degree of dilatation; the ultrasonic appearance of the renal parenchyma, including presence/absence of a kidney, echogenicity, evidence of cysts or dysplasia, cortical thickness, and corticomedullary differentiation; the presence, volume, and structure of the bladder; any evidence of dilatation elsewhere in the urinary tract; the presence of other abnormalities of the urogenital system (such as duplication) or outside the urinary tract; amniotic fluid volume; and the progression of all findings over serial evaluations (Pates & Dashe, 2006). Several diagnostic algorithms have been proposed for the evaluation of patients with prenatally detected hydronephrosis (de Kort et al., 2008; Ismaili et al., 2005; Karnak et al., 2009; Riccabona et al., 2008; Shokeir & Nijman, 2000; Yiee & Wilcox, 2008).

4.2 Postnatal diagnosis

In the neonate with a suspected urological obstruction, multiple modalities may be needed for full evaluation. Renal ultrasound and voiding cytourethrogram usually play important roles in postnatal assessment of these patients, and in some cases CT, MRI, diuretic renography, urodynamic studies, or cystoscopy may be useful.

If not detected prenatally, congenital obstructive nephropathy may present in the neonate, infant, child, adolescent or adult with poor urine output, weak urine stream, abdominal distention, palpable abdominal or flank mass, pain, incontinence, urinary tract infection, hematuria, altered serum chemistries, or as an incidental finding on imaging studies.

4.3 Prospective diagnostic and prognostic biomarkers

Many attempts have been made to identify useful diagnostic and prognostic biomarkers for congenital obstructive nephropathy. These include gestational age at diagnosis (Hutton et al., 1994); the volume of amniotic fluid (Oliveira et al., 2000; Sarhan et al., 2008); the presence of megacystis (Oliveira, et al., 2000); the appearance of the renal parenchyma on prenatal ultrasound (Morris et al., 2009; Robyr, et al., 2005; Sarhan, et al., 2008); fetal urinary sodium, calcium, β2-microglobulin, and other urinary solutes and proteins (Decramer et al., 2008; Morris et al., 2007). Additionally, pilot studies show that urine proteome analysis can identify urodynamically significant UPJ obstruction in infants with hydronephrosis with a sensitivity of 83% and a specificity of 92%, although the test had poor diagnostic accuracy in patients older than 1 year of age (Drube et al., 2010). Although several of these markers and tests show promise as diagnostic or prognostic tools, no consensus yet exists as to the best panel of biomarkers to assess congenital obstructive nephropathy.

Prenatally, the volume of amniotic fluid as well as ultrasound appearance of the bladder, urethra, and kidneys are common discriminators of the plan of care. Analysis of fetal urine can provide additional information; fetal urinary sodium less than 100 mmol/L, chloride less than 90 mmol/L, osmolality less than 210 mOsm/L, and low levels of urinary protein indicate good renal function (Shokeir & Nijman, 2000). Postnatally and in patients who present outside the neonatal period, management decisions are most frequently reliant on ultrasonography findings and other imaging modalities, coupled with serial measurements of serum creatinine. Serum creatinine is a relatively late marker of renal injury whose elevation often signals irreversible kidney damage (Nickavar et al., 2008; Sarhan et al., 2010). Nonetheless, nadir serum creatinine level is a useful and reliable prognostic indicator in patients with congenital obstructive nephropathy (Ansari et al., 2010; Bajpai et al., 2001; Warshaw et al., 1985).

5. Clinical course, management, and outcomes

The effects of fetal urinary tract obstruction on renal development, renal function, and urodynamics will be unique to each individual patient, and there may be significant clinical variability between patients thought to have similar obstructive lesions or processes. The clinical course is influenced by many factors; those intrinsic to each patient include the developmental stage at which the obstruction arises, the degree and duration of blockage, and its location. However, accurate tools to measure and determine the prognostic impact of these various factors in any individual case do not exist.

5.1 Management of congenital upper urinary tract obstruction

Regardless of the specific cause, unilateral upper urinary tract obstructive lesions rarely result in azotemia. Conservative management of these patients is often recommended, with surgery reserved for patients with clinical symptoms or declining renal function. However, over time up to 50% of patients with unilateral UPJ obstruction will meet these criteria and require surgical correction (Chertin et al., 2006). Additionally, some authors have raised concern about an increased long-term risk for hypertension as a result of ureteral obstruction, advocating for reconsideration of these conservative management approaches (Carlstrom, 2010). Relative to unilateral obstruction, bilateral upper tract obstruction or obstruction of a solitary functional kidney is far more ominous, and generally requires prompt surgical intervention and careful postsurgical management to minimize and monitor renal injury.

5.2 Natural history of lower urinary tract obstruction

Obstruction of the bladder outlet or urethra affects urologic and renal functions at all points proximal to the lesion. Extrarenal effects may also occur, primarily in the lungs due to associated oligohydramnios. The profound changes that can result are outlined in Figure 6.

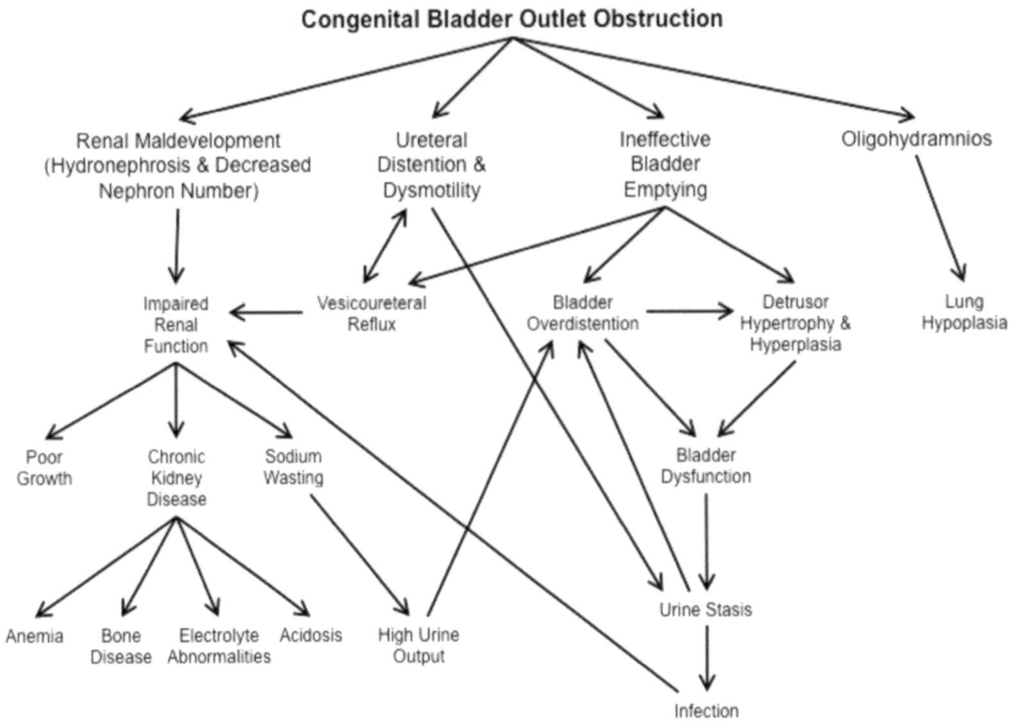

Fig. 6. Cascade of physiological consequences associated with lower urinary tract obstruction.

As many as 70% of boys with PUV develop advanced chronic or end-stage kidney disease (CKD Stage 3-5; Parkhouse et al., 1988; Reinberg et al., 1992; Roth et al., 2001; Sanna-Cherchi, et al., 2009). Those with ultrasound findings at or before 24 weeks' gestation are significantly more likely to have a poor renal outcome than children with PUV detected later in pregnancy after a normal second trimester scan (Hutton, et al., 1994). Among patients with PUV who survive the perinatal period, bladder dysfunction and nadir serum creatinine greater than 1.0 mg/dl are independent risk factors for progression to end stage renal disease (Ansari, et al., 2010; DeFoor et al., 2008). Unilateral or bilateral VUR associated with PUV may also have a significant impact on kidney function (Heikkila et al., 2009).

Long-term follow-up studies decades after treatment for PUV offer additional insight into the postnatal renal progression of this condition. Holmdahl and colleagues (2005) assessed Swedish men who were treated for PUV between 1956 and 1970. Over the 30 to 40 years between initial intervention and this follow-up assessment, the prevalence of ESRD in this population increased from 8% to 21%, and only 37% of the cohort had apparently normal renal function as adults (Holmdahl & Sillen, 2005). Kousidis et al. (2008) found that in a British cohort of patients diagnosed prenatally between 1984 and 1996, 28% died or developed ESRD and 58% had normal renal function after a mean follow-up of 17.7 years. The authors of the latter study note that for the more severely affected patients, the functional outcome may be primarily determined by the severity of intrauterine obstruction and presence of renal dysplasia and not significantly altered by early diagnosis and treatment; however, for patients with more moderate disease, long-term prognosis may be improved by prenatal diagnosis and early interventions (Kousidis, et al., 2008). Other studies have not shown a statistically significant difference in outcomes between patients with renal dysplasia and those with normal-appearing kidneys (Nickavar, et al., 2008; Ylinen et al., 2004).

5.3 Antenatal intervention

Antenatal intervention for suspected fetal obstructive nephropathy has been attempted by vesicoamniotic shunting, vesicocentesis, fetal cystoscopy, or open fetal bladder surgery. The results are variable and these methods remain controversial. A 2003 meta-analysis of the available data suggested improved perinatal survival following prenatal bladder drainage, particularly in cases with poor predicted prognoses (Clark et al., 2003). However, these procedures carry a high risk for complications including shunt malfunction or migration, urinary ascites, hemorrhage, chorioamnionitis, iatrogenic gastroschisis, premature labor, or miscarriage (Carr & Kim, 2010; Elder et al., 1987). The Percutaneous shunting in Low Urinary Tract Obstruction (PLUTO) study, a multicenter, prospective, randomized trial, was designed to systematically evaluate the prenatal and perinatal outcomes and risk/benefit ratio of *in utero* intervention for urological obstruction versus conservative management, and is currently in the data analysis phase (Kilby et al., 2007; Morris & Kilby, 2009; University of Birmingham, 2011).

5.4 Postnatal intervention

In cases where renal function is affected or threatened, surgical relief of the obstruction or diversion of the urine path is necessary. Stents, catheters, or percutaneous drains may be useful to provide temporary drainage, but long-term management requires surgery. Discussion of the variety of surgical techniques and approaches that may be implemented in the management of congenital urinary obstructions is beyond the scope of this review.

Although such surgical interventions can relieve some of the effects of congenital impairment of urine flow, many developmental and pathologic changes associated with this condition appear irreversible. Many patients with congenital obstructive nephropathy, including the majority of patients with PUV, do not have complete recovery of kidney function following postnatal intervention (Parkhouse, et al., 1988; Reinberg, et al., 1992; Roth, et al., 2001; Sanna-Cherchi, et al., 2009).

5.5 Progressive chronic kidney disease in congenital obstructive nephropathy

Given the frequency of chronic and progressive renal impairment, the importance of long-term monitoring of all patients with congenital obstructive nephropathy cannot be overemphasized. Serial measurements of renal function, periodic urinalysis, blood pressure checks, and monitoring of growth should be performed for all patients with a history of congenital urinary obstruction. Renal impairment, if detected, should be fully evaluated and managed, along with any complications of CKD such as hypertension, proteinuria, electrolyte abnormalities, metabolic acidosis, anemia, dyslipidemia, or renal bone disease. In young adult patients with congenital obstructive nephropathy and CKD, there is a strong correlation between proteinuria and rate of decline in renal function. The ItalKid Project found no benefit from angiotensin converting enzyme inhibitors (ACEi) in a population of patients with renal hypodysplasia, many of whom also had congenital obstructive nephropathy (Ardissino, 2007). However, a later study in young adults with congenital obstructive nephropathy or primary VUR with hypodysplasia indicated that ACEi can slow this decline in renal function, but impact renal outcome only when the estimated glomerular filtration rate is greater than 35 ml/min (Neild, 2009b). In patients with post-obstructive bladder dysfunction, an individualized voiding regimen designed to maintain bladder volume below a critical filling volume can stabilize deteriorating renal function (Hale et al., 2009).

5.6 End-stage kidney disease due to congenital obstructive nephropathy

For patients with congenital obstructive nephropathy who progress to ESRD, renal transplantation is generally a safe and effective therapy, with 5 year graft survival rates approximately 85% for living donor transplants and 72% for deceased donor grafts in patients with a primary diagnosis of obstructive nephropathy (NAPRTCS, 2009). Appropriate and effective management of any residual urinary tract dysfunction is critical to long-term outcomes following renal transplantation in patients with congenital obstructive nephropathy (Morita et al., 2009).

6. Experimental models of congenital obstructive nephropathy

The experimental analysis of urological obstructions dates back to antiquity. The physician Galen of Pergamon described ligature of both the ureter and the urethra in animals in the 2nd century A.D. (Galen, 1914). In the 21st century, surgical introduction of a urologic obstruction is still an important research tool. Other animal models of congenital obstructive nephropathy have been created by non-surgical approaches, including genetic manipulation and chemical induction. This review focuses on animal models for investigating the consequences of obstruction on the subsequent maturation and function of the kidneys and urinary tract. For an analysis of how mouse models have contributed to understanding ureter and bladder organogenesis from the earliest stages of development, we recommend Dr. Mendelsohn's excellent review (Mendelsohn, 2009).

6.1 Surgical models

6.1.1 Ureteral ligation/Unilateral ureteral obstruction

The vast majority of data on the progression of renal injury following urinary tract obstruction has come from experiments involving surgical ligation of a ureter, a technique known as unilateral ureteral obstruction (UUO) (Bing et al., 2003; de Souza et al., 2004; Eroglu et al., 2004; Flynn et al., 2002; Hanai et al., 2002; Klahr & Morrissey, 2002; Stanton et al., 2003; Thiruchelvam et al., 2003). Several studies have examined partial or complete ureteral ligations in embryonic rabbits, opossums, and sheep (Becker & Baum, 2006; Kitajima et al., 2010; Steinhardt et al., 1994). In these models, animals develop hydroureteronephrosis *in utero* with variable degrees of renal dysplasia depending on the timing and severity of obstruction.

The majority of investigations using UUO have employed postnatal and adult rats, mice and pigs. In these species, nephrogenesis continues for a limited period after birth (Moritz & Wintour, 1999), so postnatal ligation in these animals may have some relevance to congenital ureteral obstructions. Even though postnatal models do not reproduce the fetal environment, the delay in renal maturation in rodents versus humans permits relative comparisons of the effects of obstruction on kidney development to be made. In addition, postnatal surgical models can isolate the effects of mechanical obstruction on the developing urinary tract from parallel renal maldevelopment, a concern that often confounds analysis of genetic models of congenital obstructive nephropathy. However, many obstructive lesions that lead to congenital obstructive nephropathy in humans arise earlier in the course of renal development, or exert their effects on the kidney more gradually, than the circumstances modeled by UUO. Therefore, the precise pathophysiological applicability of this model to congenital obstructive nephropathy remains to be determined.

UUO in rodents has been shown to have profound and often irreversible effects on renal growth, maturation, and function in neonatal and adult animals. The progressive renal injury associated with UUO has been characterized as four overlapping stages: 1) interstitial inflammation, 2) tubular and myofibroblast proliferation, 3) tubular apoptosis, and 4) interstitial fibrosis (Bascands & Schanstra, 2005; Chevalier, 2006; Klahr & Morrissey, 2002). The renin-angiotensin and transforming growth factor β (TGF-β) pathways appear to play critical roles in these changes (Bascands & Schanstra, 2005; Chevalier, 2006; Esteban et al., 2004; Inazaki et al., 2004).

6.1.2 Bladder outlet obstruction models

Surgical introduction of a bladder outlet obstruction has been investigated in fetal sheep, immature guinea pigs, and young rats (Cendron et al., 1994; Kitagawa et al., 2001; Kitagawa et al., 2004; Mostwin et al., 1991; O'Connor et al., 1997). As in ureteral obstruction models, the effects of these urethral manipulations are also highly dependent on the timing and severity of the obstruction. Experimental urethral ligation resulted in a spectrum of findings ranging from minimal renal pathology to hydronephrosis, renal dysplasia, pulmonary hypoplasia and/or Potter's sequence. Unfortunately, the data on surgical models of *in utero* bladder outlet obstruction are limited by small numbers of animals, and by the lack of complementary genetic studies since many of the large animal models are not easily amenable to genetic manipulation.

6.2 Chemically-induced models

The antineoplastic anthracycline antibiotic Adriamycin has well-known teratogenic effects, and has been used in pregnant rats to generate an animal model of congenital obstructive nephropathy (Kajbafzadeh et al., 2011; Thompson et al., 1978). At Adriamycin dosages above 1.5mg/kg/d, bladder hypoplasia or agenesis occurs in all offspring, but fetal viability is low. At decreased doses, Kajbafzadeh et al. (2011) observed a high frequency of hydronephrosis with coexisting bladder anomalies and minimal fetal lethality. The kidneys of these animals demonstrated cortical thinning and cystic dilatation of collecting ducts. However, Adriamycin-treated rats display multiple extrarenal anomalies consistent with the VATER/VACTERL association, including vertebral defects, anal atresia, tracheoesophageal fistula with esophageal atresia, and radial limb dysplasia, which complicates application of this approach to modeling congenital obstructive nephropathy.

6.3 Genetic models

Although numerous genes have been postulated to play a role in the normal and abnormal development of the urinary tract, none have been shown to be directly responsible for the primary lesions associated with congenital obstructive nephropathy in humans. Even so, several mutational or transgenic rodent models of obstructive nephropathy have been described.

6.3.1 Naturally-arising mutations associated with obstructive nephropathy

Congenital progressive hydronephrosis, a hereditary condition in a mutant strain of *C57BL/6J* mice, results from a spontaneous point mutation in the aquaporin-2 gene. Affected mice produce excessive quantities of hypotonic urine, which is believed to exceed the capacity of the ureteral peristaltic machinery producing hydronephrosis, obstructive nephropathy, and death (McDill et al., 2006). Male C57BL/KsJ mice also have a high incidence of hydronephrosis, although the mechanism of this finding has not been identified (McDill, et al., 2006; Weide & Lacy, 1991). In both of these strains, hydronephrosis is not present at birth; therefore, the urological defect is hereditary, but not congenital. Genetic models that develop *in utero* obstruction include certain inbred lines of rats (Aoki et al., 2004; Fichtner et al., 1994; Miller et al., 2004) that develop unilateral UPJ obstruction. Some of these strains display minimal or no morphological change in the renal parenchyma, but one strain of Wistar rats has been shown to develop hydronephrosis, loss of renal parenchyma, tubular and ductal atrophy and dilation, and interstitial fibrosis (Seseke et al., 2000).

6.3.2 Targeted models with complex phenotypes

Mice with the targeted deletion of ADAMTS (a disintegrin and metalloproteinase with thrombospondin motifs), lysosomal membrane protein LIMP-2/LGP85, or calcineurin also develop urinary tract obstruction in the postnatal period (Chang et al., 2004; Gamp et al., 2003; Yokoyama et al., 2002). Transgenic mice over-expressing human chorionic gonadotropin develop functional urethral obstruction that is not apparent until adulthood (Rulli et al., 2003). Mice deficient in the transcription factor *Id2* (Aoki, et al., 2004; Fichtner, et al., 1994; Miller, et al., 2004) develop unilateral UPJ obstruction. Bilateral ureteral obstruction *in utero* has been reported in mice heterozygous for bone morphogenetic protein 4 (Miyazaki et al., 2000). However, each of these animal models exhibits complex urological phenotypes including renal hypoplasia, dysplasia, aplasia, ureteral tortuosity, or duplicated ureters, thereby confounding analysis due to the inextricability of the secondary effects of obstruction from primary renal maldevelopment.

Developmental urinary tract anomalies including hydronephrosis also arise from knockout of the uroplakin II or III genes and conditional knockout of homeobox gene Lim1 in the nephric duct epithelium (Hu et al., 2000; Kong et al., 2004; Pedersen et al., 2005). However, VUR is also a prominent feature in these CAKUT models, and it is not clear whether there is a true or a functional obstruction, nor what the relative contributions of reflux and obstruction to the renal phenotype are.

Mice lacking either of the two angiotensin receptors likewise develop abnormal renal phenotypes. The Agtr2 knockout has incomplete penetrance, with approximately 2-20% of mutant mice demonstrating a wide spectrum of renal and urological anomalies including UPJ stenosis or megaureter as well as multicystic dysplastic kidney, hypoplastic kidney, VUR, or duplicated ureter (Nishimura, et al., 1999). Deficiency of Agtr1 produces a renal phenotype with some features similar to that seen in complete UUO, including papillary atrophy, medullary thinning, calyceal enlargement, tubulointerstitial apoptosis, macrophage infiltration, and fibrosis. The Agtr1 mutant also demonstrates hypertrophy of the renal vasculature, a feature not seen in UUO models. There is some evidence supporting a role for Agtr1 in promoting growth and contractility of smooth muscle cells (Miyazaki & Ichikawa, 2001), but the relative contributions of primary effects of the mutation on renal development and secondary consequences of a possible functional obstruction in these mice remain unclear. Agtr1 knockout mice also display significant extrarenal abnormalities, including poor weight gain, marked hypotension, and increased frequency of ventral septal defects (Tsuchida et al., 1998).

6.3.3 Megabladder mouse

Our laboratory has identified a unique transgenic mouse model of congenital obstructive nephropathy designated the megabladder (*mgb*) mouse (Ingraham et al., 2010; Singh et al., 2007). As shown in Figure 7, these mice develop a nonfunctional, over-distended bladder due to a bladder-specific defect in smooth muscle differentiation. This leads to a functional lower urinary tract obstruction, antenatal hydronephrosis, and signs of renal failure evident shortly after birth. Male *mgb* homozygotes develop early renal insufficiency and rarely survive beyond 4-6 weeks, whereas females may live a year or longer.

Megabladder mice closely mirror the pathophysiology associated with a lower urinary tract obstruction in several key respects (Ingraham, et al., 2010; Singh, et al., 2007). *Mgb-/-* mice develop a functional obstruction of the lower urinary tract that leads to hydroureteronephrosis during embryogenesis. *Mgb-/-* mice are born with histopathological evidence of renal injury, indicating that their kidneys possess preexisting pathological changes resulting from *in utero* obstruction. The obstruction and its renal consequences develop within the uterine and fetal environment, in contrast to the postnatal timing of obstruction in UUO and many genetic models of obstructive nephropathy. *Mgb-/-* mice preferentially develop right-sided hydronephrosis reminiscent of the "pop-off" mechanism theorized in children with PUV and secondary unilateral VUR (Greenfield, et al., 1983). *Mgb-/-* mice also exhibit a variable clinical course, in much the same way that children with seemingly identical obstructive lesions may have very different clinical outcomes. Male *mgb-/-* mice can be rescued from the complications of renal failure and early demise by cutaneous vesicostomy, but of the vesicostomized animals that survive the perioperative period, approximately 40% die within the first two weeks despite a patent stoma and no apparent surgical complications. This result is reminiscent of the fact that 27% to 70% of children with PUV will have progressive CKD despite surgery (Ansari, et al., 2010; Kousidis, et al., 2008; Parkhouse, et al., 1988; Roth, et al., 2001; Sanna-Cherchi, et al., 2009). Finally, *mgb-/-* mice possess no extrarenal features to complicate their utilization as a functional model of congenital obstructive nephropathy. Taken together, these observations suggest that *mgb-/-* mice represent an excellent experimental model for the study of the pathophysiological events associated with congenital obstructive nephropathy involving the lower urinary tract.

In the kidneys of *mgb-/-* mice, fibrotic changes are observed in a distinctive pattern. Increased interstitial collagen deposition is first apparent in the renal parenchyma immediately subadjacent to the urothelium of the renal capsule, followed by the outer cortex near the renal capsule. In severe cases, fibrosis ultimately extends throughout the renal parenchyma. Altered patterns of α-smooth muscle isoactin (α-SMA), E-cadherin, TGF-β1 and connective tissue growth factor expression are also observed in *mgb-/-* kidneys, supporting a role for these pathways in the development of fibrosis associated with congenital obstructive nephropathy (Ingraham, et al., 2010). Severely affected *mgb-/-* kidneys also display several dysplastic features including alteration in the developmental distribution of WT1 and PAX2. These observations are consistent with Edith Potter's classic work suggesting that the renal pathology associated with CAKUT includes varying degrees of renal hypodysplasia (Potter, 1972). In contrast to the well-characterized UUO model of upper urinary tract obstruction, inflammation does not appear to play a prominent or early role in the pathogenesis of renal injury in the megabladder model.

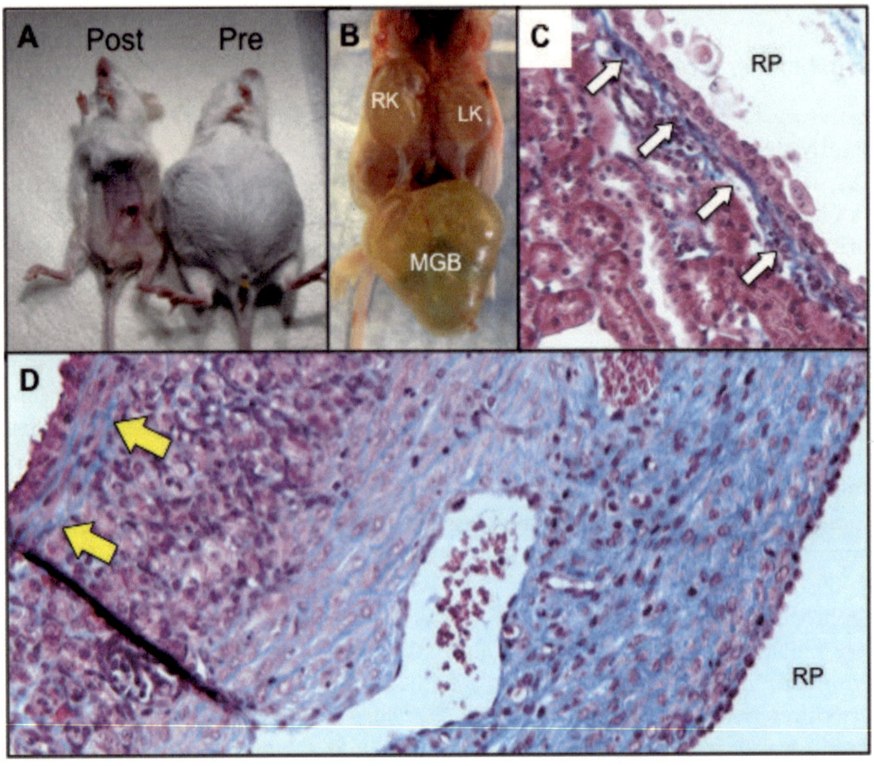

Fig. 7. Megabladder (*mgb*) mouse. **A.** Two *mgb-/-* mice, prior to (right) and immediately after (left) cutaneous vesicostomy. The mouse on the right demonstrates a massively distended abdomen secondary to the megabladder, whereas the mouse on the left demonstrates the flat belly attained with decompression of the bladder. **B.** Upon dissection and with the megabladder (MGB) reflected caudally, hydroureteronephrosis involving both kidneys (RK and LK) is apparent. **C.** Trichrome staining demonstrates a band of fibrosis (white arrows) underlying the urothelium in a mildly affected *mgb-/-* mouse. **D.** In a more severely affected kidney from a *mgb-/-* mouse, interstitial fibrosis (blue staining) extends throughout the renal medulla, and in a stripe along the outer cortex (yellow arrows) adjacent to the renal capsule.

7. Conclusion

Morbidity and mortality remain very high for patients with congenital obstructive nephropathy, with few effective therapeutic options. Clearly, additional research is needed to illuminate the cellular and molecular changes that characterize congenital obstructive nephropathy, with particular emphasis on developing reliable biomarkers and new therapeutic approaches to reduce the impact of this devastating disease. Experimental animal models of obstructive nephropathy have provided valuable information regarding renal pathogenesis and function following surgical occlusion or genetic manipulation. The continued development of new animal models of congenital obstructive nephropathy, like the *mgb* mouse, will provide increasing opportunities to identify and manipulate the key molecular pathways associated with the development of chronic renal failure, while at the same time providing an experimental platform for biomarker development and the assessment of novel therapeutic strategies.

8. Acknowledgment

We thank Dr. Andrew Schwaderer and Dr. Brian Becknell for valuable comments in drafting this manuscript, Ashley R. Carpenter for technical assistance in obtaining images of the *mgb* mouse, and our clinical colleagues at Nationwide Children's Hospital for patient cases and associated images.

9. References

Agarwal, S. (1999). Urethral valves. *BJU Int, 84*(5), 570-578.

Anderson, P. A., & Travers, A. H. (1993). Development of hydronephrosis in spina bifida patients: predictive factors and management. *Br J Urol, 72*(6), 958-961.

Ansari, M. S., Gulia, A., Srivastava, A., & Kapoor, R. (2010). Risk factors for progression to end-stage renal disease in children with posterior urethral valves. *J Pediatr Urol, 6*(3), 261-264.

Aoki, Y., Mori, S., Kitajima, K., Yokoyama, O., Kanamaru, H., Okada, K., & Yokota, Y. (2004). Id2 haploinsufficiency in mice leads to congenital hydronephrosis resembling that in humans. *Genes Cells, 9*(12), 1287-1296.

Ardissino, G., Viganò, S., Testa, S., Daccò, V., Paglialonga, F., Leoni, A., Belingheri, M., Avolio, L., Ciofani, A., Claris-Appiani, A., Cusi, D., Edefonti, A., Ammenti, A., Cecconi, M., Fede, C., Ghio, L., La Manna, A., Maringhini, S., Papalia, T., Pela, I., Pisanello, L., & Ratsch, I. M. (2007). No clear evidence of ACEi efficacy on the progression of chronic kidney disease in children with hypodysplastic nephropathy - report from the ItalKid Project database. *Nephrol Dial Transplant, 22*(9), 2525-2530.

Arena, S., Romeo, C., Borruto, F. A., Racchiusa, S., Di Benedetto, V., & Arena, F. (2009). Anterior urethral valves in children: an uncommon multipathogenic cause of obstructive uropathy. *Pediatr Surg Int, 25*(7), 613-616.

Bajpai, M., Dave, S., & Gupta, D. K. (2001). Factors affecting outcome in the management of posterior urethral valves. *Pediatr Surg Int, 17*(1), 11-15.

Bascands, J. L., & Schanstra, J. P. (2005). Obstructive nephropathy: insights from genetically engineered animals. *Kidney Int, 68*(3), 925-937.

Becker, A., & Baum, M. (2006). Obstructive uropathy. *Early Hum Dev, 82*(1), 15-22.

Bernardes, L. S., Aksnes, G., Saada, J., Masse, V., Elie, C., Dumez, Y., Lortat-Jacob, S. L., & Benachi, A. (2009). Keyhole sign: how specific is it for the diagnosis of posterior urethral valves? *Ultrasound Obstet Gynecol, 34*(4), 419-423.

Bing, W., Chang, S., Hypolite, J. A., DiSanto, M. E., Zderic, S. A., Rolf, L., Wein, A. J., & Chacko, S. (2003). Obstruction-induced changes in urinary bladder smooth muscle contractility: a role for Rho kinase. *Am J Physiol Renal Physiol, 285*(5), F990-997.

Brown, T., Mandell, J., & Lebowitz, R. L. (1987). Neonatal hydronephrosis in the era of sonography. *AJR Am J Roentgenol, 148*(5), 959-963.

Carlstrom, M. (2010). Causal link between neonatal hydronephrosis and later development of hypertension. *Clin Exp Pharmacol Physiol, 37*(2), e14-23.

Carr, M. C., & Kim, S. S. (2010). Prenatal management of urogenital disorders. *Urol Clin North Am, 37*(2), 149-158.

Cendron, M., Horton, C. E., Karim, O. M., Takishima, H., Haberlik, A., Mostwin, J. L., & Gearhart, J. P. (1994). A fetal lamb model of partial urethral obstruction: experimental protocol and results. *J Pediatr Surg, 29*(1), 77-80.

Chang, C. P., McDill, B. W., Neilson, J. R., Joist, H. E., Epstein, J. A., Crabtree, G. R., & Chen, F. (2004). Calcineurin is required in urinary tract mesenchyme for the development of the pyeloureteral peristaltic machinery. *J Clin Invest, 113*(7), 1051-1058.

Chertin, B., Pollack, A., Koulikov, D., Rabinowitz, R., Hain, D., Hadas-Halpren, I., & Farkas, A. (2006). Conservative treatment of ureteropelvic junction obstruction in children with antenatal diagnosis of hydronephrosis: lessons learned after 16 years of follow-up. *Eur Urol, 49*(4), 734-738.

Chevalier, R. L. (2006). Pathogenesis of renal injury in obstructive uropathy. *Curr Opin Pediatr, 18*(2), 153-160.

Clark, T. J., Martin, W. L., Divakaran, T. G., Whittle, M. J., Kilby, M. D., & Khan, K. S. (2003). Prenatal bladder drainage in the management of fetal lower urinary tract obstruction: a systematic review and meta-analysis. *Obstet Gynecol, 102*(2), 367-382.

de Kort, E. H., Bambang Oetomo, S., & Zegers, S. H. (2008). The long-term outcome of antenatal hydronephrosis up to 15 millimetres justifies a noninvasive postnatal follow-up. *Acta Paediatr, 97*(6), 708-713.

de Souza, G. M., Costa, W. S., Bruschini, H., & Sampaio, F. J. (2004). Morphological analysis of the acute effects of overdistension on the extracellular matrix of the rat urinary bladder wall. *Ann Anat, 186*(1), 55-59.

Decramer, S., P, Z. U. R., Wittke, S., Mischak, H., Bascands, J. L., & Schanstra, J. P. (2008). Identification of urinary biomarkers by proteomics in newborns: use in obstructive nephropathy. *Contrib Nephrol, 160*, 127-141.

DeFoor, W., Clark, C., Jackson, E., Reddy, P., Minevich, E., & Sheldon, C. (2008). Risk factors for end stage renal disease in children with posterior urethral valves. *J Urol, 180*(4 Suppl), 1705-1708.

Drube, J., Zurbig, P., Schiffer, E., Lau, E., Ure, B., Gluer, S., Kirschstein, M., Pape, L., Decramer, S., Bascands, J. L., Schanstra, J. P., Mischak, H., & Ehrich, J. H. (2010). Urinary proteome analysis identifies infants but not older children requiring pyeloplasty. *Pediatric nephrology, 25*(9), 1673-1678.

Eagle, J. F., Jr., & Barrett, G. S. (1950). Congenital deficiency of abdominal musculature with associated genitourinary abnormalities: A syndrome. Report of 9 cases. *Pediatrics, 6*(5), 721-736.

Elder, J. S., Duckett, J. W., Jr., & Snyder, H. M. (1987). Intervention for fetal obstructive uropathy: has it been effective? *Lancet, 2*(8566), 1007-1010.

Eroglu, E., Kucukhuseyin, C., Ayik, B., Dervisoglu, S., Emir, H., & Danismend, N. (2004). Changes in the threshold voltage and alterations of smooth-muscle physiology after bladder outlet obstruction. *Eur J Pediatr Surg, 14*(1), 39-44.

Esteban, V., Lorenzo, O., Ruperez, M., Suzuki, Y., Mezzano, S., Blanco, J., Kretzler, M., Sugaya, T., Egido, J., & Ruiz-Ortega, M. (2004). Angiotensin II, via AT1 and AT2 receptors and NF-kappaB pathway, regulates the inflammatory response in unilateral ureteral obstruction. *J Am Soc Nephrol, 15*(6), 1514-1529.

Ewalt, D. H., & Bauer, S. B. (1996). Pediatric neurourology. *Urol Clin North Am, 23*(3), 501-509.

Farnham, S. B., Adams, M. C., Brock, J. W., 3rd, & Pope, J. C. t. (2005). Pediatric urological causes of hypertension. *J Urol, 173*(3), 697-704.

Fichtner, J., Boineau, F. G., Lewy, J. E., Sibley, R. K., Vari, R. C., & Shortliffe, L. M. (1994). Congenital unilateral hydronephrosis in a rat model: continuous renal pelvic and bladder pressures. *J Urol, 152*(2 Pt 2), 652-657.

Flynn, B. J., Mian, H. S., Cera, P. J., Kabler, R. L., Mowad, J. J., Cavanaugh, A. H., & Rothblum, L. I. (2002). Early molecular changes in bladder hypertrophy due to bladder outlet obstruction. *Urology, 59*(6), 978-982.

Galen. (1914). *On the Natural Faculties* (A. J. Brock, Trans.). New York: G. P. Putnam's Sons.

Gamp, A. C., Tanaka, Y., Lullmann-Rauch, R., Wittke, D., D'Hooge, R., De Deyn, P. P., Moser, T., Maier, H., Hartmann, D., Reiss, K., Illert, A. L., von Figura, K., & Saftig, P. (2003). LIMP-2/LGP85 deficiency causes ureteric pelvic junction obstruction, deafness and peripheral neuropathy in mice. *Hum Mol Genet, 12*(6), 631-646.

Gillenwater, J. Y., Westervelt, F. B., Jr., Vaughan, E. D., Jr., & Howards, S. S. (1975). Renal function after release of chronic unilateral hydronephrosis in man. *Kidney Int, 7*(3), 179-186.

Gimpel, C., Masioniene, L., Djakovic, N., Schenk, J. P., Haberkorn, U., Tonshoff, B., & Schaefer, F. (2010). Complications and long-term outcome of primary obstructive megaureter in childhood. *Pediatric nephrology, 25*(9), 1679-1686.

Gonzalez, R., De Filippo, R., Jednak, R., & Barthold, J. S. (2001). Urethral atresia: long-term outcome in 6 children who survived the neonatal period. *J Urol, 165*(6 Pt 2), 2241-2244.

Greenfield, S. P., Hensle, T. W., Berdon, W. E., & Wigger, H. J. (1983). Unilateral vesicoureteral reflux and unilateral nonfunctioning kidney associated with posterior urethral valves--a syndrome? *J Urol, 130*(4), 733-738.

Gupta, D. K., & Srinivas, M. (2000). Congenital anterior urethral diverticulum in children. *Pediatr Surg Int, 16*(8), 565-568.

Hale, J. M., Wood, D. N., Hoh, I. M., Neild, G. H., Bomanji, J. B., Chu, A., & Woodhouse, C. R. (2009). Stabilization of renal deterioration caused by bladder volume dependent obstruction. *J Urol, 182*(4 Suppl), 1973-1977.

Hanai, T., Ma, F. H., Matsumoto, S., Park, Y. C., & Kurita, T. (2002). Partial outlet obstruction of the rat bladder induces a stimulatory response on proliferation of the bladder smooth muscle cells. *Int Urol Nephrol, 34*(1), 37-42.

Heikkila, J., Rintala, R., & Taskinen, S. (2009). Vesicoureteral reflux in conjunction with posterior urethral valves. *J Urol, 182*(4), 1555-1560.

Herndon, C. D., & Casale, A. J. (2002). Early second trimester intervention in a surviving infant with postnatally diagnosed urethral atresia. *J Urol, 168*(4 Pt 1), 1532-1533.

Holmdahl, G., & Sillen, U. (2005). Boys with posterior urethral valves: outcome concerning renal function, bladder function and paternity at ages 31 to 44 years. *J Urol, 174*(3), 1031-1034; discussion 1034.

Hosgor, M., Karaca, I., Ulukus, C., Ozer, E., Ozkara, E., Sam, B., Ucan, B., Kurtulus, S., Karkiner, A., & Temir, G. (2005). Structural changes of smooth muscle in congenital ureteropelvic junction obstruction. *J Pediatr Surg, 40*(10), 1632-1636.

Hu, P., Deng, F. M., Liang, F. X., Hu, C. M., Auerbach, A. B., Shapiro, E., Wu, X. R., Kachar, B., & Sun, T. T. (2000). Ablation of uroplakin III gene results in small urothelial plaques, urothelial leakage, and vesicoureteral reflux. *J Cell Biol, 151*(5), 961-972.

Hutton, K. A., Thomas, D. F., Arthur, R. J., Irving, H. C., & Smith, S. E. (1994). Prenatally detected posterior urethral valves: is gestational age at detection a predictor of outcome? *J Urol, 152*(2 Pt 2), 698-701.

Inazaki, K., Kanamaru, Y., Kojima, Y., Sueyoshi, N., Okumura, K., Kaneko, K., Yamashiro, Y., Ogawa, H., & Nakao, A. (2004). Smad3 deficiency attenuates renal fibrosis, inflammation,and apoptosis after unilateral ureteral obstruction. *Kidney Int, 66*(2), 597-604.

Ingraham, S. E., Saha, M., Carpenter, A., Robinson, M., Ismail, I., Singh, S., Hains, D., Robinson, M., Hirselj, D. A., Koff, S., Bates, C. M., & McHugh, K. M. (2010). Pathogenesis of renal injury in the Megabladder mouse: A genetic model of congenital obstructive nephropathy. *Pediatr Res, 68*, 500-507.

Ismaili, K., Hall, M., Donner, C., Thomas, D., Vermeylen, D., & Avni, F. E. (2003). Results of systematic screening for minor degrees of fetal renal pelvis dilatation in an unselected population. *Am J Obstet Gynecol, 188*(1), 242-246.

Ismaili, K., Hall, M., Piepsz, A., Alexander, M., Schulman, C., & Avni, F. E. (2005). Insights into the pathogenesis and natural history of fetuses with renal pelvis dilatation. *Eur Urol, 48*(2), 207-214.

Kajbafzadeh, A. M., Javan-Farazmand, N., Motamedi, A., Monajemzadeh, M., & Amini, E. (2011). The optimal dose of Adriamycin to create a viable rat model potentially applicable to congenital obstructive uropathy. *J Pediatr Surg, 46*(8), 1544-1549.

Karnak, I., Woo, L. L., Shah, S. N., Sirajuddin, A., & Ross, J. H. (2009). Results of a practical protocol for management of prenatally detected hydronephrosis due to ureteropelvic junction obstruction. *Pediatr Surg Int, 25*(1), 61-67.

Kilby, M., Khan, K., Morris, K., Daniels, J., Gray, R., Magill, L., Martin, B., Thompson, P., Alfirevic, Z., Kenny, S., Bower, S., Sturgiss, S., Anumba, D., Mason, G., Tydeman, G., Soothill, P., Brackley, K., Loughna, P., Cameron, A., Kumar, S., & Bullen, P. (2007). PLUTO trial protocol: percutaneous shunting for lower urinary tract obstruction randomised controlled trial. *BJOG, 114*(7), 904-905, e901-904.

King, L. R. (1985). Posterior urethral valves. In P. Kelalis, L. R. King & A. B. Belman (Eds.), *Clinical Pediatric Urology* (2nd ed., pp. 527-558). Philadelphia W. B. Saunders.

Kitagawa, H., Pringle, K. C., Koike, J., Zuccollo, J., & Nakada, K. (2001). Different phenotypes of dysplastic kidney in obstructive uropathy in fetal lambs. *J Pediatr Surg, 36*(11), 1698-1703.

Kitagawa, H., Pringle, K. C., Koike, J., Zuccollo, J., Sato, Y., Sato, H., Fujiwaki, S., Odanaka, M., & Nakada, K. (2004). The early effects of urinary tract obstruction on glomerulogenesis. *J Pediatr Surg, 39*(12), 1845-1848.

Kitajima, K., Aoba, T., Pringle, K. C., Seki, Y., Zuccollo, J., Koike, J., Chikaraishi, T., & Kitagawa, H. (2010). Bladder development following bladder outlet obstruction in fetal lambs: optimal timing of fetal therapy. *J Pediatr Surg, 45*(12), 2423-2430.

Klahr, S., & Morrissey, J. (2002). Obstructive nephropathy and renal fibrosis. *Am J Physiol Renal Physiol, 283*(5), F861-875.

Kong, X. T., Deng, F. M., Hu, P., Liang, F. X., Zhou, G., Auerbach, A. B., Genieser, N., Nelson, P. K., Robbins, E. S., Shapiro, E., Kachar, B., & Sun, T. T. (2004). Roles of uroplakins in plaque formation, umbrella cell enlargement, and urinary tract diseases. *J Cell Biol, 167*(6), 1195-1204.

Kousidis, G., Thomas, D. F., Morgan, H., Haider, N., Subramaniam, R., & Feather, S. (2008). The long-term outcome of prenatally detected posterior urethral valves: a 10 to 23-year follow-up study. *BJU Int, 102*(8), 1020-1024.

McDill, B. W., Li, S. Z., Kovach, P. A., Ding, L., & Chen, F. (2006). Congenital progressive hydronephrosis (cph) is caused by an S256L mutation in aquaporin-2 that affects its phosphorylation and apical membrane accumulation. *Proc Natl Acad Sci U S A, 103*(18), 6952-6957.

Mendelsohn, C. (2009). Using mouse models to understand normal and abnormal urogenital tract development. *Organogenesis, 5*(1), 306-314.

Miller, J., Hesse, M., Diemer, T., Haenze, J., Knerr, I., Rascher, W., & Weidner, W. (2004). Congenital unilateral ureteropelvic junction obstruction of the rat: a useful animal model for human ureteropelvic junction obstruction? *Urology, 63*(1), 190-194.

Miyazaki, Y., & Ichikawa, I. (2001). Role of the angiotensin receptor in the development of the mammalian kidney and urinary tract. *Comp Biochem Physiol A Mol Integr Physiol, 128*(1), 89-97.

Miyazaki, Y., Oshima, K., Fogo, A., Hogan, B. L., & Ichikawa, I. (2000). Bone morphogenetic protein 4 regulates the budding site and elongation of the mouse ureter. *J Clin Invest, 105*(7), 863-873.

Morita, K., Iwami, D., Hotta, K., Shimoda, N., Miura, M., Watarai, Y., Hoshii, S., Obikane, K., Nakashima, T., Sasaki, S., & Nonomura, K. (2009). Pediatric kidney transplantation is safe and available for patients with urological anomalies as well as those with primary renal diseases. *Pediatr Transplant, 13*(2), 200-205.

Moritz, K. M., & Wintour, E. M. (1999). Functional development of the meso- and metanephros. *Pediatr Nephrol, 13*(2), 171-178.

Morris, R. K., & Kilby, M. D. (2009). An overview of the literature on congenital lower urinary tract obstruction and introduction to the PLUTO trial: percutaneous shunting in lower urinary tract obstruction. *Aust N Z J Obstet Gynaecol, 49*(1), 6-10.

Morris, R. K., Malin, G. L., Khan, K. S., & Kilby, M. D. (2009). Antenatal ultrasound to predict postnatal renal function in congenital lower urinary tract obstruction: systematic review of test accuracy. *BJOG, 116*(10), 1290-1299.

Morris, R. K., Quinlan-Jones, E., Kilby, M. D., & Khan, K. S. (2007). Systematic review of accuracy of fetal urine analysis to predict poor postnatal renal function in cases of congenital urinary tract obstruction. *Prenat Diagn, 27*(10), 900-911.

Mostwin, J. L., Karim, O. M., van Koeveringe, G., & Brooks, E. L. (1991). The guinea pig as a model of gradual urethral obstruction. *J Urol, 145*(4), 854-858.

NAPRTCS. (2009). North American Pediatric Renal Transplant Cooperative Study (NAPRTCS) 2008 annual report. October 16, 2011, Available from https://web.emmes.com/study/ped/annlrept/Archiveannlrept.html

Neild, G. H. (2009a). What do we know about chronic renal failure in young adults? I. Primary renal disease. *Pediatr Nephrol, 24*(10), 1913-1919.

Neild, G. H. (2009b). What do we know about chronic renal failure in young adults? II. Adult outcome of pediatric renal disease. *Pediatr Nephrol, 24*(10), 1921-1928.

Nickavar, A., Otoukesh, H., & Sotoudeh, K. (2008). Validation of initial serum creatinine as a predictive factor for development of end stage renal disease in posterior urethral valves. *Indian J Pediatr, 75*(7), 695-697.

Nishimura, H., Yerkes, E., Hohenfellner, K., Miyazaki, Y., Ma, J., Hunley, T. E., Yoshida, H., Ichiki, T., Threadgill, D., Phillips, J. A., 3rd, Hogan, B. M., Fogo, A., Brock, J. W., 3rd, Inagami, T., & Ichikawa, I. (1999). Role of the angiotensin type 2 receptor gene in congenital anomalies of the kidney and urinary tract, CAKUT, of mice and men. *Mol Cell, 3*(1), 1-10.

O'Connor, L. T., Jr., Vaughan, E. D., Jr., & Felsen, D. (1997). In vivo cystometric evaluation of progressive bladder outlet obstruction in rats. *J Urol, 158*(2), 631-635.

Oliveira, E. A., Diniz, J. S., Cabral, A. C., Pereira, A. K., Leite, H. V., Colosimo, E. A., & Vilasboas, A. S. (2000). Predictive factors of fetal urethral obstruction: a multivariate analysis. *Fetal Diagn Ther, 15*(3), 180-186.

Pagon, R. A., Smith, D. W., & Shepard, T. H. (1979). Urethral obstruction malformation complex: a cause of abdominal muscle deficiency and the "prune belly". *J Pediatr, 94*(6), 900-906.

Parkhouse, H. F., Barratt, T. M., Dillon, M. J., Duffy, P. G., Fay, J., Ransley, P. G., Woodhouse, C. R., & Williams, D. I. (1988). Long-term outcome of boys with posterior urethral valves. *Br J Urol, 62*(1), 59-62.

Pates, J. A., & Dashe, J. S. (2006). Prenatal diagnosis and management of hydronephrosis. *Early Hum Dev, 82*(1), 3-8.

Payabvash, S., Kajbafzadeh, A. M., Tavangar, S. M., Monajemzadeh, M., & Sadeghi, Z. (2007). Myocyte apoptosis in primary obstructive megaureters: the role of decreased vascular and neural supply. *J Urol, 178*(1), 259-264; discussion 264.

Pedersen, A., Skjong, C., & Shawlot, W. (2005). Lim 1 is required for nephric duct extension and ureteric bud morphogenesis. *Dev Biol, 288*(2), 571-581.

Pohl, H. G., Joyce, G. F., Wise, M., & Cilento, B. G., Jr. (2007). Vesicoureteral reflux and ureteroceles. *J Urol, 177*(5), 1659-1666.

Potter, E. L. (1972). *Normal and abnormal development of the kidney*. Chicago: Year Book Medical Publishers, Inc.

Rawat, J., Khan, T. R., Singh, S., Maletha, M., & Kureel, S. (2009). Congenital anterior urethral valves and diverticula: diagnosis and management in six cases. *Afr J Paediatr Surg, 6*(2), 102-105.

Reinberg, Y., Chelimsky, G., & Gonzalez, R. (1993). Urethral atresia and the prune belly syndrome. Report of 6 cases. *Br J Urol, 72*(1), 112-114.

Reinberg, Y., de Castano, I., & Gonzalez, R. (1992). Prognosis for patients with prenatally diagnosed posterior urethral valves. *J Urol, 148*(1), 125-126.

Reinberg, Y., Shapiro, E., Manivel, J. C., Manley, C. B., Pettinato, G., & Gonzalez, R. (1991). Prune belly syndrome in females: a triad of abdominal musculature deficiency and anomalies of the urinary and genital systems. *J Pediatr, 118*(3), 395-398.

Riccabona, M., Avni, F. E., Blickman, J. G., Dacher, J. N., Darge, K., Lobo, M. L., & Willi, U. (2008). Imaging recommendations in paediatric uroradiology: minutes of the ESPR workgroup session on urinary tract infection, fetal hydronephrosis, urinary tract ultrasonography and voiding cystourethrography, Barcelona, Spain, June 2007. *Pediatr Radiol, 38*(2), 138-145.

Riedmiller, H., Androulakakis, P., Beurton, D., Kocvara, R., & Gerharz, E. (2001). EAU guidelines on paediatric urology. *Eur Urol, 40*(5), 589-599.

Robyr, R., Benachi, A., Daikha-Dahmane, F., Martinovich, J., Dumez, Y., & Ville, Y. (2005). Correlation between ultrasound and anatomical findings in fetuses with lower urinary tract obstruction in the first half of pregnancy. *Ultrasound Obstet Gynecol, 25*(5), 478-482.

Roth, K. S., Carter, W. H., Jr., & Chan, J. C. (2001). Obstructive nephropathy in children: long-term progression after relief of posterior urethral valve. *Pediatrics, 107*(5), 1004-1010.

Routh, J. C., Huang, L., Retik, A. B., & Nelson, C. P. (2010). Contemporary Epidemiology and Characterization of Newborn Males with Prune Belly Syndrome. *Urology, 76*(1), 44-48.

Rulli, S. B., Ahtiainen, P., Makela, S., Toppari, J., Poutanen, M., & Huhtaniemi, I. (2003). Elevated steroidogenesis, defective reproductive organs, and infertility in transgenic male mice overexpressing human chorionic gonadotropin. *Endocrinology, 144*(11), 4980-4990.

Sanna-Cherchi, S., Ravani, P., Corbani, V., Parodi, S., Haupt, R., Piaggio, G., Innocenti, M. L., Somenzi, D., Trivelli, A., Caridi, G., Izzi, C., Scolari, F., Mattioli, G., Allegri, L., & Ghiggeri, G. M. (2009). Renal outcome in patients with congenital anomalies of the kidney and urinary tract. *Kidney Int, 76*(5), 528-533.

Sarhan, O., El-Dahshan, K., & Sarhan, M. (2010). Prognostic value of serum creatinine levels in children with posterior urethral valves treated by primary valve ablation. *J Pediatr Urol, 6*(1), 11-14.

Sarhan, O., Zaccaria, I., Macher, M. A., Muller, F., Vuillard, E., Delezoide, A. L., Sebag, G., Oury, J. F., Aigrain, Y., & El-Ghoneimi, A. (2008). Long-term outcome of prenatally detected posterior urethral valves: single center study of 65 cases managed by primary valve ablation. *J Urol, 179*(1), 307-312.

Seseke, F., Thelen, P., Hemmerlein, B., Kliese, D., Zoller, G., & Ringert, R. H. (2000). Histologic and molecular evidence of obstructive uropathy in rats with hereditary congenital hydronephrosis. *Urol Res, 28*(2), 104-109.

Shokeir, A. A., & Nijman, R. J. (2000). Antenatal hydronephrosis: changing concepts in diagnosis and subsequent management. *BJU Int, 85*(8), 987-994.

Singh, S., Robinson, M., Nahi, F., Coley, B., Robinson, M. L., Bates, C. M., Kornacker, K., & McHugh, K. M. (2007). Identification of a unique transgenic mouse line that develops megabladder, obstructive uropathy, and renal dysfunction. *J Am Soc Nephrol, 18*(2), 461-471.

Sozubir, S., Lorenzo, A. J., Twickler, D. M., Baker, L. A., & Ewalt, D. H. (2003). Prenatal diagnosis of a prolapsed ureterocele with magnetic resonance imaging. *Urology, 62*(1), 144.

Stanton, M. C., Clement, M., Macarak, E. J., Zderic, S. A., & Moreland, R. S. (2003). Partial bladder outlet obstruction alters Ca2+ sensitivity of force, but not of MLC phosphorylation, in bladder smooth muscle. *Am J Physiol Renal Physiol, 285*(4), F703-710.

Steinhardt, G. F., Salinas-Madrigal, L., deMello, D., Farber, R., Phillips, B., & Vogler, G. (1994). Experimental ureteral obstruction in the fetal opossum: histologic assessment. *J Urol, 152*(6 Pt 1), 2133-2138.

Strand, W. R. (2004). Initial management of complex pediatric disorders: prunebelly syndrome, posterior urethral valves. *Urol Clin North Am, 31*(3), 399-415, vii.

Straub, E., & Spranger, J. (1981). Etiology and pathogenesis of the prune belly syndrome. *Kidney Int, 20*(6), 695-699.

Thiruchelvam, N., Wu, C., David, A., Woolf, A. S., Cuckow, P. M., & Fry, C. H. (2003). Neurotransmission and viscoelasticity in the ovine fetal bladder after in utero bladder outflow obstruction. *Am J Physiol Regul Integr Comp Physiol, 284*(5), R1296-1305.

Thompson, D. J., Molello, J. A., Strebing, R. J., & Dyke, I. L. (1978). Teratogenicity of adriamycin and daunomycin in the rat and rabbit. *Teratology, 17*(2), 151-157.

Tsuchida, S., Matsusaka, T., Chen, X., Okubo, S., Niimura, F., Nishimura, H., Fogo, A., Utsunomiya, H., Inagami, T., & Ichikawa, I. (1998). Murine double nullizygotes of the angiotensin type 1A and 1B receptor genes duplicate severe abnormal phenotypes of angiotensinogen nullizygotes. *J Clin Invest, 101*(4), 755-760.

University of Birmingham. (2011). PLUTO (Percutaneous shunting in Lower Urinary Tract Obstruction) trial home page. October 12, 2011, Available from http://www.pluto.bham.ac.uk

van Gool, J. D., Dik, P., & de Jong, T. P. (2001). Bladder-sphincter dysfunction in myelomeningocele. *Eur J Pediatr, 160*(7), 414-420.

Vidal, I., Heloury, Y., Ravasse, P., Lenormand, L., & Leclair, M. D. (2009). Severe bladder dysfunction revealed prenatally or during infancy. *J Pediatr Urol, 5*(1), 3-7.

Warshaw, B. L., Hymes, L. C., Trulock, T. S., & Woodard, J. R. (1985). Prognostic features in infants with obstructive uropathy due to posterior urethral valves. *J Urol, 133*(2), 240-243.

Weide, L. G., & Lacy, P. E. (1991). Hereditary hydronephrosis in C57BL/KsJ mice. *Lab Anim Sci, 41*(5), 415-418.

Wiesel, A., Queisser-Luft, A., Clementi, M., Bianca, S., & Stoll, C. (2005). Prenatal detection of congenital renal malformations by fetal ultrasonographic examination: an analysis of 709,030 births in 12 European countries. *Eur J Med Genet, 48*(2), 131-144.

Woodhouse, C. R., Ransley, P. G., & Innes-Williams, D. (1982). Prune belly syndrome--report of 47 cases. *Arch Dis Child, 57*(11), 856-859.

Woodward, M., & Frank, D. (2002). Postnatal management of antenatal hydronephrosis. *BJU Int, 89*(2), 149-156.

Woolf, A. S., & Thiruchelvam, N. (2001). Congenital obstructive uropathy: its origin and contribution to end-stage renal disease in children. *Adv Ren Replace Ther, 8*(3), 157-163.

Yiee, J., & Wilcox, D. (2008). Management of fetal hydronephrosis. *Pediatr Nephrol, 23*(3), 347-353.

Ylinen, E., Ala-Houhala, M., & Wikstrom, S. (2004). Prognostic factors of posterior urethral valves and the role of antenatal detection. *Pediatr Nephrol, 19*(8), 874-879.

Yokoyama, H., Wada, T., Kobayashi, K., Kuno, K., Kurihara, H., Shindo, T., & Matsushima, K. (2002). A disintegrin and metalloproteinase with thrombospondin motifs (ADAMTS)-1 null mutant mice develop renal lesions mimicking obstructive nephropathy. *Nephrol Dial Transplant, 17 Suppl 9*, 39-41.

Yoon, J. Y., Kim, J. C., Hwang, T. K., Yoon, M. S., & Park, Y. H. (1998). Collagen studies for pediatric ureteropelvic junction obstruction. *Urology, 52*(3), 494-497.

2

Association Between Haemoglobin Variability and Clinical Outcomes in Chronic Kidney Disease

Roshini Malasingam, David W. Johnson and Sunil V. Badve
Princess Alexandra Hospital, Brisbane, QLD,
Australasian Kidney Trials Network, The University of Queensland, Brisbane, QLD,
Australia

1. Introduction

Anaemia is a common complication of chronic kidney disease (CKD). The underlying physiology related to anaemia in CKD is secondary to reduction in endogenous erythropoietin as the glomerular filtration rate (GFR) declines. The introduction of erythropoiesis stimulating agents (ESA) has revolutionized the management of anaemia in CKD, leading to substantial reductions in the blood transfusion requirements, improvement in energy and physical function and small improvements in health-related quality of life (Clement et. al., 2009; Eschbach et. al., 1987; Gandra et. al., 2010). Targeting higher haemoglobin with ESA therapy has been associated with increased risks of stroke, vascular access thrombosis, hypertension and possibly death (Badve et. al., 2011; Besarab et. al., 1998; Palmer et. al., 2010; Pfeffer et. al., 2009; Phrommintikul et. al., 2007; Singh et. al., 2006). The current KDOQI Clinical Practice Guideline recommends a haemoglobin target of 11-12g/dL. However, a substantial proportion of non-dialysis and dialysis CKD patients exhibit fluctuations in the haemoglobin levels, also known as haemoglobin variability. There is an emerging body of evidence demonstrating an association between haemoglobin variability and mortality in CKD patients treated with ESAs. Maintaining haemoglobin levels within narrow target range remains a major challenge in clinical practice. The aim of this chapter is to review the definition, prevalence, risk factors of haemoglobin variability, and its impact on survival, provide recommendations where possible and suggest directions for future research.

2. Haemoglobin variability

2.1 Definition

The definition of haemoglobin variability is not entirely clear and various studies have used different definitions. Intra-individual haemoglobin variability is defined as the fluctuation of haemoglobin above or below (Kalantar-Zadeh & Aronoff 2009) *or* even within the target range over time. Methods to quantify haemoglobin variability are summarised below.

1. Standard deviation of the differences between observed haemoglobin values and haemoglobin slope which represents the mean haemoglobin change over time (Yang et. al., 2007).

2. Intra-individual standard deviation of 3-month haemoglobin rolling average (Lacson et. al., 2003).
3. Using 3 haemoglobin groups (above/below/within the target) for each of the 6 consecutive monthly haemoglobin values, classification of all patients into 6 groups: (i) consistently low, (ii) consistently high, (iii) consistently within the target range, (iv) low amplitude fluctuation with low haemoglobin values (all-6 mo with low or target-range haemoglobin values), (v) low amplitude fluctuation with high haemoglobin values (all-6 mo with high or target-range haemoglobin values), and (vi) high amplitude fluctuation with high haemoglobin values (low, high and target-range haemoglobin values within 6-mo period) (Ebben et. al., 2006).
4. Time-in-target haemoglobin range (De Nicola et. al., 2007).
5. Determining velocity (or deflection) of haemoglobin change by averaging slopes between successive haemoglobin values (Lau et. al., 2010).
6. Change in haemoglobin in 6-mo above and below the reference range (based on the median change in haemoglobin in 6-mo) (Regidor et. al., 2006).

2.2 Prevalence

Haemoglobin variability is common not only in patients with end-stage kidney disease (ESKD) on dialysis, but also in CKD patients who are not yet on dialysis (non-dialysis CKD). The reported prevalence of haemoglobin variability in non-dialysis CKD patients varies between 61 to 86% (Boudville et. al., 2009; Minutolo et. al., 2009). On the other hand, 82 to 90% of ESKD patients on dialysis exhibit haemoglobin variability (Ebben et al., 2006; Eckardt et. al., 2010; Gilbertson et. al., 2009).

3. Risk factors

3.1 ESA therapy

Requirement of ESA for the treatment of anaemia in CKD is a major risk factor for haemoglobin variability. In a study involving 6,165 non-dialysis CKD patients, only 47% of patients who were not treated with any ESAs demonstrated fluctuations in haemoglobin (Boudville et al., 2009). However, 73% of patients who were already treated with ESAs experienced haemoglobin variability. This prevalence further increased to 77% among individuals who were commenced on ESAs as a new therapy. Patients treated with ESA therapy for a longer duration were less likely to have haemoglobin variability. Each 3-mo increment in the duration of ESA therapy decreased the risk of haemoglobin variability by 6%. In a study involving 5,037 ESKD patients on haemodialysis, the risk of developing haemoglobin variability was more than twice in patients on ESAs, compared to those not on ESAs (Eckardt et al., 2010). These findings suggest that the *need* of ESA rather than ESA therapy *per se* leads to haemoglobin variability (See Table 1).

There is increased interest in studying the effect of various anaemia management protocols on haemoglobin variability. Patel and colleagues studied the effect of route of administration of erythropoietin on haemoglobin variability in a post hoc analysis of a randomised controlled trial involving 157 prevalent ESKD patients on dialysis (Patel et. al., 2009). Over a follow up of 24-weeks, compared to patients treated with intravenous erythropoietin, those treated with subcutaneous erythropoietin were more likely to have (i)

Factors related to ESA therapy
Route of administration
Long *versus* short acting ESA
Responsiveness to the first dose of ESA
Haemoglobin before initiation of ESA
Iron supplementation
Frequency of the ESA dose adjustments
Magnitude of the ESA dose adjustments
Patient-level factors
Age
Gender
Body mass index
Incident *versus* prevalent dialysis
Comorbid conditions
Number and duration of hospitalisation
Use of catheter as haemodialysis vascular access
Facility-level anaemia management protocols
Proportion of patients prescribed ESAs
Frequency of haemoglobin monitoring
Frequency of ESA dose monitoring
Wider range of target haemoglobin
Higher upper target range of haemoglobin

Table 1. List of possible factors affecting haemoglobin variability

haemoglobin concentrations outside the target range for more weeks (13.9 ± 4.7 weeks versus 12.5 ± 5 weeks, p=0.04) and (ii) higher standard deviation of haemoglobin (0.84 ± 0.35 versus 0.74 ± 0.27, p=0.01). Interestingly, in one report, the risk of developing haemoglobin variability was greater with long-acting ESAs (Boudville et al., 2009). De Nicola and colleagues did not find any association between long-acting ESAs versus erythropoietin and haemoglobin variability (De Nicola et al., 2007). However, they observed that baseline haemoglobin level, first dose of ESA and initial iron supplementation were directly associated with the length of time-in-target haemoglobin.

Depending on the 6-group classification based on the highest and lowest categories of haemoglobin, Gilbertson and colleagues reported that patients in the low-intermediate group received high doses of erythropoietin and more blood transfusions (Gilbertson et al., 2009). Minutolo and colleagues found that haemoglobin variability was associated with responsiveness to the first dose of erythropoietin (Minutolo et al., 2009). They also observed that a change of erythropoietin dosage occurred less frequently than expected in spite of regular follow up visits. Therefore, they concluded that lack of adjustment of erythropoietin dosage can lead to haemoglobin variability. However, their data on the effect of frequency and magnitude of adjustment of erythropoietin dosage on haemoglobin stabilisation is less clear. In a post hoc analysis of a randomised controlled trial involving 154 ESKD patients on haemodialysis, more frequent adjustments of erythropoietin dosage as well as larger changes of erythropoietin dosage were associated with haemoglobin variability (Lau et al., 2010).

Using data from the Dialysis Outcomes and Practice Patterns Study (DOPPS) involving 26,510 patients, Pisoni and colleagues studied the associations between facility-level anaemia management practices and facility-level haemoglobin standard deviations (Pisoni et. al., 2011). This study identified factors that decreased haemoglobin variability which include reviewing ESA dose at least twice a week and checking haemoglobin levels on a weekly basis. There was also less haemoglobin variability in facilities with a greater percentage of patients prescribed an ESA likely related to better anaemia management with the introduction of an ESA and fewer patients outside the target haemoglobin concentration. The factors that were more likely associated with haemoglobin variability were: facilities with a wider target haemoglobin range, higher upper target haemoglobin, and ESA administration by subcutaneous route (compared to intravenous route).

3.2 Patient-level factors

Various studies have reported that young age is a risk factor for haemoglobin variability (De Nicola et al., 2007; Eckardt et al., 2010). Boudville and colleagues reported that the odds of haemoglobin variability decreased by 11% with each 10-yr increment in age (Boudville et al., 2009). A few studies have reported that women were more likely to have fluctuations in the haemoglobin concentration (Ebben et al., 2006; Gilbertson et. al., 2008). In a study of 119 non-dialysis CKD patients, male gender was directly associated with increased time-in-target haemoglobin (De Nicola et al., 2007).

Eckardt and colleagues studied the magnitude and frequency of haemoglobin variability as a quantitative index by integrating the area under the curve (AUC) between measured haemoglobin values and the mean haemoglobin concentration (Eckardt et al., 2010). High degree of haemoglobin variability was defined as AUC >50th percentile. The mean body mass index (BMI) was lowest in the highest quartile of AUC. On multivariate logistic regression, BMI 25 to 30 kg/m^2 and >30 kg/m^2 were independently associated with decreased odds of haemoglobin variability compared to the reference category of BMI 18 to 25 kg/m^2. Similarly, Lau and colleagues also observed less positive deflection of haemoglobin in heavier patients (Lau et al., 2010).

There is an excess burden of comorbid conditions in CKD, leading to erythropoietin hyporesponsiveness. In an observational study involving 152,846 ESKD patients on haemodialysis, Ebben and colleagues reported that having 2 or more comorbid conditions, 6 or more days of hospitalisation, and occurrence of infectious hospitalisations were independently associated with haemoglobin variability (Ebben et al., 2006).

Eckardt and colleagues found that incident dialysis vintage, change in haemodialysis vascular access, use of catheter for haemodialysis, haemoglobin lower than 11 g/dL, use of angiotensin-converting enzyme inhibitor or angiotensin receptor blocker, and hospitalisation were positively associated with an increased risk of haemoglobin variability (Eckardt et al., 2010). Also, patients treated with an ESA were twice likely to experience hemoglobin variability than those not treated with an ESA. As expected, higher serum albumin concentration was negatively associated with haemoglobin variability. Interestingly, history of cardiovascular disease was negatively associated with haemoglobin variability. Furthermore, the investigators did not find any association of C-reactive protein and leukocyte count with haemoglobin variability. The reasons for these findings are not entirely clear, but this study included a highly selected cohort in whom complete data on monthly haemoglobin values for 6 mo and medications were available, raising a possibility of selection bias. Similarly, Lau and colleagues also found a positive association between catheter use and haemoglobin variability; and a negative association with high baseline haemoglobin (Lau et al., 2010).

Weinhandl and colleagues studied the risk factors for haemoglobin variability in Medicare haemodialysis patients (Weinhandl et. al., 2011). The study cohort included 3 groups of haemodialysis patients: historical prevalent (prevalent on July 1, 1996; n=78,602), contemporary prevalent (prevalent on July 1, 2006; n= 133,246), and incident (January 1, 2005 - June 30, 2006; n=24,999). In both the prevalent groups, the presence of all comorbid conditions, except hepatic disease, was associated with greater haemoglobin variability. These conditions included atherosclerotic heart disease, congestive heart failure, arrhythmia and other cardiac diseases, cerebrovascular disease, peripheral vascular disease, cancer, chronic obstructive pulmonary disease, diabetes and gastrointestinal bleeding. In the incident group, the presence of cerebrovascular disease, peripheral vascular disease, chronic obstructive pulmonary disease, diabetes and gastrointestinal bleeding were associated with haemoglobin variability. In all 3 groups, cumulative hospital days and number of months with haemoglobin <10 g/dL were positively associated with haemoglobin variability. Similar findings have been reported by Gilbertson and colleagues (Gilbertson et al., 2009).

3.3 Facility-level factors

Pisoni and colleagues studied facility-level risk factors for haemoglobin variability in 26,510 haemoglobin patients from 930 facilities in 12 countries using the DOPPS data (Pisoni et al., 2011). Haemoglobin variability was not associated with the number of haemodialysis patients per facility. However, larger differences in mean facility-level haemoglobin standard deviation were seen between countries. The mean age was nearly 2 years younger in the highest quartile of facility-level haemoglobin standard deviation than the lowest quartile. The investigators found that BMI, neutrophil count, and prevalence of psychiatric disorders and hepatitis C were higher in facilities with higher facility-level haemoglobin standard deviation. They also observed a positive association between haemoglobin variability and increased proportion of patients in a facility with parathyroid hormone level >450 pg/mL. Furthermore, the investigators reported a strong correlation (r =0.56) between facility-level haemoglobin standard deviation and within-patient haemoglobin standard deviation. These findings suggest that the results of this facility-level study could be generalised to an individual patient.

4. Association between haemoglobin variability and mortality

An emerging body of evidence suggests that haemoglobin variability is associated with increased risk of all-cause death in both non-dialysis CKD and ESKD patients. Boudville and colleagues found an association between haemoglobin variability and death not only in non-dialysis CKD patients treated with ESAs (n=1,823), but also in those who were not on ESAs (n=3,143) (Boudville et al., 2009). For each 1 g/L increase in the residual standard deviation, HR (95%CI) for patients on ESA throughout the study and those who were not receiving ESA were 1.02 (1.01 to 1.04) and 1.03 (1.02 to 1.05), respectively. The analysis of the pooled data from these 2 groups showed similar results. Compared to patients with haemoglobin levels consistently within the target range, those with low amplitude fluctuation with low haemoglobin values (HR 1.62, 95%CI 1.36 to 1.94) and high amplitude fluctuation (HR 1.57, 95%CI 1.24 to 1.98) were at increased risk of all-cause mortality.

Minutolo and colleagues reported that longer time with haemoglobin within the target range of 11 to 13 g/dL was associated with decreased risk of renal death (defined as a composite endpoint of all-cause death on dialysis or after kidney transplantation) (Minutolo et al., 2009).

In a study involving 34,963 haemodialysis patients who were enrolled in the Fresenius Medical Care database in 1996, Yang and colleagues reported that the risk of all-cause mortality increased proportionately with haemoglobin variability (Yang et al., 2007). The hazard ratio and 95% confidence intervals (CI) per 0.50 g/dL, 0.75 g/dL, 1.00 g/dL, and 1.50 g/dL increases in haemoglobin variability were 1.15 (1.10 to 1.20), 1.24 (1.16 to 1.32), 1.33 (1.22 to 1.45), and 1.53 (1.35 to 1.75), respectively.

Gilbertson and colleagues found that out of 6 categories of haemoglobin variability (categorized as low <11g/dL, intermediate 11 - 12.5g/dL & high >12.5g/dL and further divided into low-low, intermediate-intermediate, high-high, low-intermediate, intermediate-high, low-high), patients in the low-high and low-intermediate groups experienced an increased risk of death compared with those in the intermediate-intermediate group (Gilbertson et al., 2008). The HR and 95%CI for the low-high and low-intermediate groups were 1.19 (1.10 to 1.28) and 1.44 (1.33 to 1.56), respectively. Although this categorization broadly identifies patients with stable hemoglobin and either low or high amplitude fluctuations in hemoglobin, it assumes a unidirectional and linear change in hemoglobin.

Lau and colleagues measured haemoglobin variability as rate of haemoglobin change: average positive-only (positive haemoglobin deflections) and average negative-only (negative haemoglobin deflections) (Lau et al., 2010). While negative haemoglobin deflections were not associated with mortality risk (HR 1.07, 95% CI 0.94 to 1.21 per g/L/week), rapid rise in haemoglobin was associated increased risk (HR 1.23, 95% CI 1.03 to 1.48 per g/L/week).

Regidor and colleagues analysed a cohort of 58,058 prevalent haemodialysis patients from the DaVita dialysis organisation (Regidor et al., 2006). Compared to patients whose haemoglobin remain unchanged during the first 6 mo of the 2-year cohort study period, the risks of all-cause and cardiovascular mortality were significantly higher in patients with reduction in haemoglobin by more than 1.50 g/dL/quarter. In the fully-adjusted model (adjusted for demographic characteristics, comorbidities, smoking, dialysis dose, nutritional status, iron studies, doses of ESAs and iron), there was no association observed with increment in haemoglobin and mortality. However, decrease in hemoglobin was associated with increased mortality. While this study described an association between change in hemoglobin per quarter and mortality, it did not specifically study an association between hemoglobin variability and mortality.

Pisoni and colleagues reported mortality outcomes using haemoglobin variability at the facility-level using the DOPPS database (Pisoni et al., 2011). In the adjusted model, the HR for every 0.5 g/dL higher facility-level haemoglobin standard deviation was 1.08 (95% CI 1.02 to 1.15). Compared to the reference category of the lowest quartile of facility-level haemoglobin standard deviation, the HR (95% CI) for the 2nd, 3rd and 4th quartiles were 1.08 (1.10 to 1.34), 1.15 (1.35 to 1.69) and 1.19 (1.04 to 1.37), respectively. As previously mentioned, the facility-level haemoglobin standard deviation correlated well with within-patient haemoglobin standard deviation.

Not all studies have demonstrated a positive association between haemoglobin variability and death in CKD. Eckardt and colleagues studied the effect of haemoglobin variability on mortality using 5 definitions: within-patient standard deviation, residual standard deviation, time-in-target haemoglobin, amplitudes of fluctuation, and AUC (Eckardt et al., 2010). In the adjusted Cox regression model, haemoglobin variability was not a statistically significant factor in all 5 methods, except for the group of patients with low amplitude fluctuations with low haemoglobin levels (HR 1.74, 95%CI 1.00 to 3.04). However, 95% confidence intervals were very wide and the lower 95% confidence interval was 1.00. Thus, although this association was statistically significant, it was weak.

Brunelli and colleagues included a retrospective cohort of 6,644 incident patients who commenced haemodialysis between 2004 and 2005 from the Fresenius Medical Centre database (Brunelli et. al., 2008). In contrast to their 1996 cohort study results (Yang et al., 2007), the association between haemoglobin variability and mortality was not statistically significant. The unadjusted and adjusted HR (95%CI) for were 0.96 (0.81 to 1.14) and 1.11 (0.92 to 1.33), respectively. The discrepancy in these analyses may be explained by the addition of a large number of variables in the Cox regression model for the 2004-2005 cohort as more data were available. Consequently, when the analysis was restricted using the same limited variables as in the 1996 cohort study; the association achieved statistical significance with a HR of 1.22 (1.01 to 1.48). Although the investigators have attempted to adjust for known variables, the possibility of residual confounding could not be excluded. The complexity of these statistical models makes interpretation of the results difficult, particularly when the different statistical methods or approaches did not generate robust or consistent findings.

Weinhandl and colleagues reported the association between haemoglobin variability and all-cause mortality using 3 Cox proportional hazards regression models (Weinhandl et al., 2011). In the case-mix-adjusted model, the HR (95%CI) for the contemporary prevalent, historical prevalent and incident groups for 1 g/dL haemoglobin variability were 1.27 (1.24 to 1.31), 1.32 (1.27 to 1.38) and 1.08 (1.03 to 1.13), respectively. In the comorbid condition-adjusted model, haemoglobin variability was associated with increased risk of death in both the prevalent groups with a HR of 1.07 (1.04 to 1.10) in the contemporary prevalent group and 1.10 (1.06 to 1.15) in the historical prevalent group. However, there was no statistically significant association in the incident group (HR 1.03, 95%CI 0.98 to 1.09). In the expanded comorbid condition-adjusted model, the statistically significant association was limited only to the historical prevalent group (HR 1.07, 95%CI 1.03 to 1.12). Haemoglobin variability was not associated with increased risk of death in either the contemporary prevalent (HR 1.02, 95%CI 0.99 to 1.05) or incident groups (HR 1.01, 95%CI 0.95 to 1.06). These findings suggest that the association between haemoglobin variability and mortality was weak in this study and was sensitive to adjustment for concurrent disease severity.

5. Management of haemoglobin variability

Since the introduction of ESAs, most of the clinical trials with ESA therapy have focused on haemoglobin targets in CKD patients. There is a shortage of clinical trials studying the optimal strategy for haemoglobin monitoring in patients treated with ESAs and interventions to reduce haemoglobin variability.

Ho and colleagues conducted an observational case-control study of unselected ESKD patients on haemodialysis (Ho et. al., 2010). Patients served as their own control. They compared 2x/month laboratory haemoglobin measurements and use of a computerised algorithm to analyse 12x/month monitoring of Crit-line haemoglobin measurements. They found that haemoglobin variability, measured by the mean standard deviation of the residuals, significantly improved during the phase of frequent haemoglobin monitoring. However, this was not a randomised controlled trial. Also, the sample size was small and it was an unblinded study in a single-centre. Nonetheless, the study highlights the importance of frequent monitoring of haemoglobin as it may provide an opportunity to titrate the ESA dose early.

Gaweda and colleagues conducted a case-controlled observational study in which 49 ESKD patients on haemodialysis were included (Gaweda et. al., 2010). The investigators measured haemoglobin using Crit-line at various intervals: twice weekly or 8x/mo, once weekly or 4x/mo, every 2 weeks or 2x/mo and every 4 weeks or 1x/mo. They also calculated the haemoglobin estimation error as a root mean-squared difference between the observed and estimated haemoglobin and compared it with the measurement error. They found that the most accurate haemoglobin estimation was achieved with twice weekly haemoglobin sampling, although it exceeded the accuracy of the measurement device. Twice and once weekly haemoglobin measurements were found to be optimal in 31% and 45% patients, respectively. This was also a single-centre study with a small sample size.

These two studies highlight the paucity of evidence in the area of management of haemoglobin variability. Considering the cost and possible amount of blood loss associated with frequent hemoglobin monitoring, currently available evidence is not sufficient to make any clinical practice recommendations.

6. Future research

There is substantial heterogeneity in the haematological response to ESAs. Although the factors underpinning ESA-hyporesponsiveness are well characterised, those contributing to haemoglobin variability are poorly understood. Future studies should include prospective and systematic data collection to evaluate these factors. Investigations should also be carried out to develop a single and uniformly accepted method to measure haemoglobin variability that is clinically relevant and reproducible, since there is no consensus on a single method for the measurement of haemoglobin variability.

The data on the effect of haemoglobin variability on mortality are conflicting. This could be due to several reasons. Firstly, most of the data originates from retrospective and observational studies. Secondly, the studies are arbitrarily limited to sampling during 6 month periods where monthly haemoglobin values for each month were available. This cross-sectional nature of the study does not reflect long-term fluctuations in haemoglobin values. Thirdly, due to highly selective nature of the study cohorts, sampling bias could be potentially introduced. Most of these studies had a very short follow up period ranging from 6 months to 18 months. Furthermore, different statistical models have demonstrated inconsistent and non-reproducible results due considerable between-study variation in the covariates included in the adjusted models. Therefore, the exact nature and quantification of the effect of haemoglobin variability on mortality is still poorly understood.

Future studies should be designed carefully and conducted prospectively to define the exact magnitude of the effect of haemoglobin variability on mortality. They should also include a greater breadth and depth of the CKD patient populations since dialysis studies have not included patients receiving peritoneal dialysis and studies involving non-dialysis CKD patients have been very limited.

Most of the current data is merely hypothesis generating. Therefore, well designed and adequately powered randomised controlled trials are needed to determine the optimal frequency of haemoglobin monitoring along with a cost-effective analysis. Further trials are required to define the optimal strategy of frequency and magnitude of ESA and iron dose changes, and study their possible interactions with concurrent acute illness and the presence of comorbid conditions.

7. Summary

Haemoglobin variability is highly prevalent in both non-dialysis and dialysis CKD patients. The factors contributing to haemoglobin variability are not entirely clear. However, the currently available evidence has identified the following factors: younger age, female gender, low body mass index, the presence of comorbid conditions, and the use of ESA and less frequent monitoring of haemoglobin. There is conflicting evidence on the effect of haemoglobin variability on mortality with some studies demonstrating a strong association and others showing no association with mortality. A few small prospective observational studies have found that frequent monitoring of haemoglobin may reduce short-term haemoglobin variability, although the optimal frequency of haemoglobin monitoring is yet to be defined. Evidence-based treatment strategies cannot be currently recommended due to a lack of high quality data. In conclusion, maintaining haemoglobin within a target range continues to pose a challenge to clinicians. Further research is urgently needed in this insufficiently researched field.

8. Acknowledgment

Professor David Johnson is a recipient of consultancy fees, research grants, travel sponsorships and speakers' honoraria from Amgen, Roche and Janssen-Cilag. He is a recipient of consultancy fees from Sandoz and is a co-investigator on industry-sponsored research by Amgen, Roche and Janssen-Cilag. He is currently supported by a Queensland Government Health Research Fellowship. Other authors do not have any conflicts of interest to declare.

9. References

Badve, S. V., Hawley, C. M. , & Johnson, D. W. (2011). Is the problem with the vehicle or the destination? Does high-dose ESA or high haemoglobin contribute to poor outcomes in CKD? *Nephrology (Carlton),* Vol.16, No.2, pp. 144-153

Besarab, A., Bolton, W. K., Browne, J. K., Egrie, J. C., Nissenson, A. R., Okamoto, D. M., Schwab, S. J. , & Goodkin, D. A. (1998). The effects of normal as compared with low hematocrit values in patients with cardiac disease who are receiving hemodialysis and epoetin. *N Engl J Med,* Vol.339, No.9, pp. 584-590

Boudville, N. C., Djurdjev, O., Macdougall, I. C., de Francisco, A. L., Deray, G., Besarab, A., Stevens, P. E., Walker, R. G., Urena, P., Inigo, P., Minutolo, R., Haviv, Y. S., Yeates, K., Aguera, M. L., MacRae, J. M. , & Levin, A. (2009). Hemoglobin variability in nondialysis chronic kidney disease: examining the association with mortality. *Clin J Am Soc Nephrol,* Vol.4, No.7, pp. 1176-1182

Brunelli, S. M., Lynch, K. E., Ankers, E. D., Joffe, M. M., Yang, W., Thadhani, R. I. , & Feldman, H. I. (2008). Association of hemoglobin variability and mortality among contemporary incident hemodialysis patients. *Clin J Am Soc Nephrol,* Vol.3, No.6, pp. 1733-1740

Clement, F. M., Klarenbach, S., Tonelli, M., Johnson, J. A. , & Manns, B. J. (2009). The impact of selecting a high hemoglobin target level on health-related quality of life for patients with chronic kidney disease: a systematic review and meta-analysis. *Arch Intern Med,* Vol.169, No.12, pp. 1104-1112

De Nicola, L., Conte, G., Chiodini, P., Cianciaruso, B., Pota, A., Bellizzi, V., Tirino, G., Avino, D., Catapano, F. , & Minutolo, R. (2007). Stability of target hemoglobin levels during the first year of epoetin treatment in patients with chronic kidney disease. *Clin J Am Soc Nephrol,* Vol.2, No.5, pp. 938-946

Ebben, J. P., Gilbertson, D. T., Foley, R. N. , & Collins, A. J. (2006). Hemoglobin level variability: associations with comorbidity, intercurrent events, and hospitalizations. *Clin J Am Soc Nephrol,* Vol.1, No.6, pp. 1205-1210

Eckardt, K. U., Kim, J., Kronenberg, F., Aljama, P., Anker, S. D., Canaud, B., Molemans, B., Stenvinkel, P., Schernthaner, G., Ireland, E., Fouqueray, B. , & Macdougall, I. C. (2010). Hemoglobin variability does not predict mortality in European hemodialysis patients. *J Am Soc Nephrol,* Vol.21, No.10, pp. 1765-1775

Eschbach, J. W., Egrie, J. C., Downing, M. R., Browne, J. K. , & Adamson, J. W. (1987). Correction of the anemia of end-stage renal disease with recombinant human erythropoietin. Results of a combined phase I and II clinical trial. *N Engl J Med,* Vol.316, No.2, pp. 73-78

Gandra, S. R., Finkelstein, F. O., Bennett, A. V., Lewis, E. F., Brazg, T. , & Martin, M. L. (2010). Impact of erythropoiesis-stimulating agents on energy and physical function in nondialysis CKD patients with anemia: a systematic review. *Am J Kidney Dis,* Vol.55, No.3, pp. 519-534

Gaweda, A. E., Nathanson, B. H., Jacobs, A. A., Aronoff, G. R., Germain, M. J. , & Brier, M. E. (2010). Determining optimum hemoglobin sampling for anemia management from every-treatment data. *Clin J Am Soc Nephrol,* Vol.5, No.11, pp. 1939-1945

Gilbertson, D. T., Peng, Y., Bradbury, B., Ebben, J. P. , & Collins, A. J. (2009). Hemoglobin level variability: anemia management among variability groups. *Am J Nephrol,* Vol.30, No.6, pp. 491-498

Gilbertson, D. T., Ebben, J. P., Foley, R. N., Weinhandl, E. D., Bradbury, B. D. , & Collins, A. J. (2008). Hemoglobin level variability: associations with mortality. *Clin J Am Soc Nephrol,* Vol.3, No.1, pp. 133-138

Ho, W. R., Germain, M. J., Garb, J., Picard, S., Mackie, M. K., Bartlett, C. , & Will, E. J. (2010). Use of 12x/month haemoglobin monitoring with a computer algorithm reduces haemoglobin variability. *Nephrol Dial Transplant,* Vol.25, No.8, pp. 2710-2714

Kalantar-Zadeh, K. & Aronoff, G. R. (2009). Hemoglobin variability in anemia of chronic kidney disease. *J Am Soc Nephrol,* Vol.20, No.3, pp. 479-487

Lacson, E., Jr., Ofsthun, N. , & Lazarus, J. M. (2003). Effect of variability in anemia management on hemoglobin outcomes in ESRD. *Am J Kidney Dis,* Vol.41, No.1, pp. 111-124

Lau, J. H., Gangji, A. S., Rabbat, C. G. , & Brimble, K. S. (2010). Impact of haemoglobin and erythropoietin dose changes on mortality: a secondary analysis of results from a randomized anaemia management trial. *Nephrol Dial Transplant,* Vol.25, No.12, pp. 4002-4009

Minutolo, R., Chiodini, P., Cianciaruso, B., Pota, A., Bellizzi, V., Avino, D., Mascia, S., Laurino, S., Bertino, V., Conte, G. , & De Nicola, L. (2009). Epoetin therapy and hemoglobin level variability in nondialysis patients with chronic kidney disease. *Clin J Am Soc Nephrol,* Vol.4, No.3, pp. 552-559

Palmer, S. C., Navaneethan, S. D., Craig, J. C., Johnson, D. W., Tonelli, M., Garg, A. X., Pellegrini, F., Ravani, P., Jardine, M., Perkovic, V., Graziano, G., McGee, R., Nicolucci, A., Tognoni, G. , & Strippoli, G. F. (2010). Meta-analysis: erythropoiesis-stimulating agents in patients with chronic kidney disease. *Ann Intern Med,* Vol.153, No.1, pp. 23-33

Patel, T., Hirter, A., Kaufman, J., Keithi-Reddy, S. R., Reda, D. , & Singh, A. (2009). Route of epoetin administration influences hemoglobin variability in hemodialysis patients. *Am J Nephrol,* Vol.29, No.6, pp. 532-537

Pfeffer, M. A., Burdmann, E. A., Chen, C. Y., Cooper, M. E., de Zeeuw, D., Eckardt, K. U., Feyzi, J. M., Ivanovich, P., Kewalramani, R., Levey, A. S., Lewis, E. F., McGill, J. B., McMurray, J. J., Parfrey, P., Parving, H. H., Remuzzi, G., Singh, A. K., Solomon, S. D. , & Toto, R. (2009). A trial of darbepoetin alfa in type 2 diabetes and chronic kidney disease. *N Engl J Med,* Vol.361, No.21, pp. 2019-2032

Phrommintikul, A., Haas, S. J., Elsik, M. , & Krum, H. (2007). Mortality and target haemoglobin concentrations in anaemic patients with chronic kidney disease treated with erythropoietin: a meta-analysis. *Lancet,* Vol.369, No.9559, pp. 381-388

Pisoni, R. L., Bragg-Gresham, J. L., Fuller, D. S., Morgenstern, H., Canaud, B., Locatelli, F., Li, Y., Gillespie, B., Wolfe, R. A., Port, F. K. , & Robinson, B. M. (2011). Facility-level interpatient hemoglobin variability in hemodialysis centers participating in the Dialysis Outcomes and Practice Patterns Study (DOPPS): Associations with mortality, patient characteristics, and facility practices. *Am J Kidney Dis,* Vol.57, No.2, pp. 266-275

Regidor, D. L., Kopple, J. D., Kovesdy, C. P., Kilpatrick, R. D., McAllister, C. J., Aronovitz, J., Greenland, S. , & Kalantar-Zadeh, K. (2006). Associations between changes in hemoglobin and administered erythropoiesis-stimulating agent and survival in hemodialysis patients. *J Am Soc Nephrol,* Vol.17, No.4, pp. 1181-1191

Singh, A. K., Szczech, L., Tang, K. L., Barnhart, H., Sapp, S., Wolfson, M. , & Reddan, D. (2006). Correction of anemia with epoetin alfa in chronic kidney disease. *N Engl J Med,* Vol.355, No.20, pp. 2085-2098

Weinhandl, E. D., Peng, Y., Gilbertson, D. T., Bradbury, B. D. , & Collins, A. J. (2011). Hemoglobin variability and mortality: confounding by disease severity. *Am J Kidney Dis,* Vol.57, No.2, pp. 255-265

Yang, W., Israni, R. K., Brunelli, S. M., Joffe, M. M., Fishbane, S. , & Feldman, H. I. (2007). Hemoglobin variability and mortality in ESRD. *J Am Soc Nephrol,* Vol.18, No.12, pp. 3164-3170

3

Complexity of Differentiating Cerebral-Renal Salt Wasting from SIADH, Emerging Importance of Determining Fractional Urate Excretion

John K. Maesaka, Louis Imbriano,
Shayan Shirazian and Nobuyuki Miyawaki
*Department of Medicine, Winthrop-University Hospital, Mineola, NY,
SUNY Medical School, Stony Brook, NY,
USA*

1. Introduction

The current approach to the diagnosis and treatment of hyponatremia is in a state of flux, largely because of an unresolved controversy regarding the relative prevalence of the syndrome of inappropriate secretion of antidiuretic hormone (SIADH) and cerebral salt wasting, or preferably renal salt wasting (RSW). The recent awareness that symptoms are now being attributed to even mild hyponatremia has led to recommendations to treat virtually all hyponatremics. (Arief et al, 1976; Berl et al, 2010; Decaux, 2006, 2009; Gankam Kegne et al, 2008; Hoorn et al, 2009; Renneboog et al, 2006; Sterns et al,2009; Schrier, 2010) This tendency to treat even mild hyponatremia introduces an urgency to resolve the diagnostic dilemma of differentiating two syndromes, SIADH and RSW, with divergent therapeutic goals, to water-restrict in SIADH or administer salt and water in RSW. We propose to define RSW by supporting data and review the pathophysiology of RSW, the derivation and evolution of the controversy over the relative prevalence of SIADH and RSW, and methods to differentiate SIADH from RSW. We will also review the emerging value of determining fractional excretion (FE) of urate in the evaluation of patients with hyponatremia by emphasizing our recent observations in reset osmostat, identify conditions that predispose to RSW, amplify the possibility that RSW might exist in patients with an increased FEurate without hyponatremia and propose an algorithm where FEurate is central to the evaluation of hyponatremia. We will also advocate and hopefully justify changing the designation, cerebral salt wasting, to renal salt wasting, and briefly discuss different strategies to treat hyponatremia.

2. Definition of RSW

In our view, RSW is most accurately defined as, "extracellular volume (ECV) depletion due to a renal sodium transport abnormality with or without high urinary sodium concentration (UNa), presence of hyponatremia or cerebral disease and normal renal, adrenal and thyroid function". (Maesaka et al, 2009) We will provide data to support our contention that UNa can be low in RSW, and how RSW can occur in normonatremic patients and in patients without cerebral disease. Although an increased FEurate has been demonstrated in a number of patients with RSW, we will withhold including FEurate to our definition of RSW until there are more confirmatory data.

2.1 Pathophysiology of RSW

RSW starts with a disease entity that appears to induce production of a natriuretic factor(s) that inhibits mainly proximal tubule sodium transport and possibly other solutes such as urate. Depending on the balance between the severity of the sodium transport defect and sodium intake, ECV depletion of varying magnitude ensues. The patient will first enter a stage of negative sodium balance, which will stimulate the renin-angiotensin aldosterone system, reduce atrial/brain natriuretic peptide (A/BNP), alter glomerular hemodynamics and possibly activate neural factors that attempt to decrease sodium excretion. (Abuelo, 2007) In some, a combination of inadequate sodium intake and profound inhibition of tubule sodium transport can lead to severe, symptomatic ECV depletion that is manifested as postural hypotension, unsteady gait, and postural somnolence, dizziness and slurred speech. (Gutierrez et al, 2007; Maesaka et al, 1990, 2007; Wijdicks et al, 1985) A more common scenario is a milder defect in sodium transport and mild ECV depletion that cannot be appreciated unless we refine our ability to diagnose RSW accurately. There are, therefore, different degrees of volume depletion that depend on the severity of the inhibition of renal sodium transport and salt and water intake. The true prevalence of RSW, therefore, cannot be appreciated until we refine methods of determining ECV accurately by simple methods or develop other as yet unidentified methods of defining RSW. Moreover, because SIADH and RSW typically present with hyponatremia, high urine osmolality and UNa, these overlapping features of RSW and SIADH and divergent therapeutic goals of each syndrome introduce an urgency to differentiate one syndrome from the other to achieve these opposing therapeutic goals.

The volume-depleted subject must reach an equilibrated state of sodium balance, otherwise a sustained negative sodium balance will result in total loss of body sodium and collapse of the vascular system. Sodium excretion and UNa can thus be low, if sodium intake is low. (Maesaka et al, 2007) A similar sequence of negative sodium balance followed by equilibration has been noted for SIADH. (Jaenike et al, 1961) The increase in water reabsorption maintains ECV at high normal and increases ANP levels, which can cause natriuresis by multiple factors. (de Zeeuw et al, 1992)

Interestingly, plasma renin in RSW can be variable depending on sodium intake, whereas plasma aldosterone tends to be increased irrespective of sodium intake when volume depleted. (Bitew et al, 2009; Maesaka et al, 2007) In this scenario, we noted increased plasma renin in a patient with RSW while on a low sodium intake. The decrease in sodium delivery to the distal tubule stimulated COX2 activity and increased plasma renin. (Traynor et al, 1999) On the other hand, a salt wasting patient on a normal sodium intake had higher sodium delivery to the distal tubule by virtue of an underlying decrease in proximal tubule sodium transport that failed to increase COX2 activity and maintained normal plasma renin, while being volume depleted. (Bitew et al, 2009; Traynor et al, 1999)

In contrast to SIADH, when ADH production fails to respond to conventional volume and osmolar stimuli, there is appropriate stimulation of ADH production in RSW by ECV depletion. The volume stimulus for ADH production is more potent than the osmolar effect on ADH production, so a volume depleted patient continues to increase ADH production, increase free water reabsorption and decrease serum sodium and osmolality. (Robertson & Ganguly, 1986) Administration of saline in our patient with RSW eliminated the volume stimulus for ADH production to allow the coexisting hypoosmolality of plasma to inhibit ADH production to indeterminate levels, thus decreasing urine osmolality, increase free water excretion and increase serum sodium, figure 1.

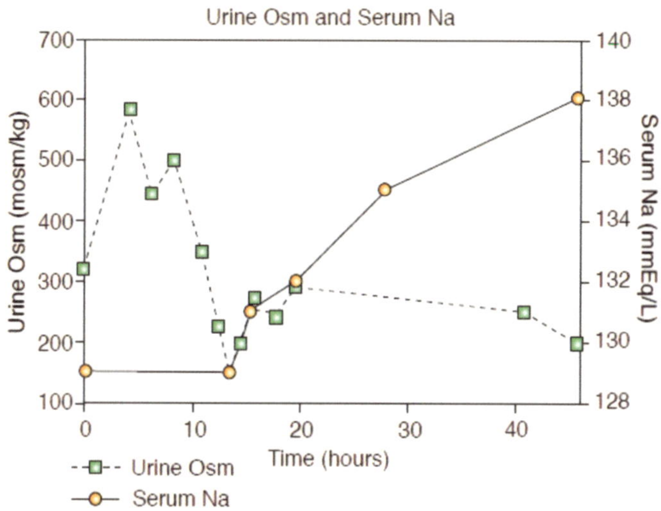

Fig. 1. Urine osmolality and serum sodium concentration during saline infusion at 125 ml/hr. over 48 hour period. Note dilution of urine 13 hours after initiation of saline, at which time a previously increased plasma ADH was not detectable, appropriate AD secretion. See text. (reproduced with permission from publisher)

This appropriate increase in plasma ADH in a patient with unequivocal RSW illustrates this important physiologic difference between RSW and SIADH. (Maesaka et al, 2007, 2009) As noted earlier, the task of clinically determining whether the increase in plasma ADH levels are appropriate or inappropriate rests solely on differences in ECV, since both present with hyponatremia, high urine osmolality and UNa. Our reliance on the assessment of ECV becomes critical in differentiating SIADH from RSW. Our inability to assess this critical parameter remains central to the unresolved controversy regarding the prevalence of SIADH and RSW. (Maesaka et al, 2009, 1999; Oh & Carroll, 1999; Singh et al, 2002).

2.2 Natriuretic factor(s) in RSW

Atrial or brain natriuretic peptide (A/BNP) has been frequently mentioned as a possible cause of the salt wasting in RSW. (Ellison & Berl, 2007; Palmer, 2003) A/BNP has been reported to be increased in patients with subarachnoid hemorrhage (SAH), a condition that has been shown to have a high prevalence for RSW, but it has also been reported to be increased in a non salt wasting syndrome such as SIADH and salt-retaining conditions such as congestive heart failure. (Burnett et al, 1986; Fichman et al, 1974; Wijdicks et al, 1991) The low normal ANP level in RSW is consistent with the volume-depleted state and strongly argues against any role of ANP in salt wasting. (Maesaka et al, 2007, Vogel, 1963)

ANP increases GFR, decreases renal blood flow and blood pressure and increases sodium excretion by the increase in GFR and inhibition of sodium transport in the proximal and distal tubule. ANP responds to changes in intravascular volume and would be lower in volume depleted states such as RSW. (Maesaka et al, 2007) The contribution of ANP in maintaining sodium homeostasis has not been clearly established, being considered by some to have no role as compared to others who feel ANP does contribute to sodium balance. (de Zeeuw et al, 1992).

The infusion of BNP into normal subjects increased GFR, decreased renal plasma flow, increased urine flow and sodium excretion, and inhibited plasma renin without affecting blood pressure, angiotensin II or aldosterone levels. There was evidence for inhibition of proximal tubule and larger inhibition of distal sodium transport. (Jensen, 1998) There is questionable relevance of these findings to RSW because A/BNP responds to changes in intravascular volume and are, thus, lower in RSW. (Maesaka et al, 2007; Vogel, 1963) We favor a natriuretic factor that does not have characteristics of A/BNP that is evident in plasma and urine of patients with evidence for RSW, see below.

We infused plasma from patients with neurosurgical and Alzheimer's diseases (AD) with increased FEurate and normonatremia into rats, and demonstrated a significant increase in FElithium and FENa, suggesting that a natriuretic factor(s) had a predominant effect on proximal tubule sodium transport. (Maesaka et al, 1993, 1993) Blood pressure and GFR remained unchanged from baseline and from controls throughout the study. Since lithium transport follows sodium transport on a one to one basis in the proximal tubule in the absence of nonelectrolyte solutes such as mannitol, the significant increase in FElithium from 22.3 and 27.2% in control animals to 36.6 and 41.7% in neurosurgical and AD patients, respectively, indicates that the same fraction of filtered sodium escaped reabsorption in the proximal tubule. (Dorhout Mees,1990; Leyssac et al, 1990; Maesaka et al 1993, 1993) This increase in distal delivery of sodium only increased FENa significantly from control values of 0.3 and 0.33% to 0.59 and 0.63% in rats infused with plasma of neurosurgical and AD, respectively, indicating that the distal tubule had actually increased distal sodium reabsorption from control values of 22.0 and 26.87% to 36.01 and 41.07% of the filtered sodium. (Maesaka et al, 1993, 1993) The significant increase in FENa indicated a net sodium loss in animals infused with plasma of neurosurgical and AD. An unresolved question is whether the increase in the distal delivery of sodium exceeded the capacity of the distal tubule to transport sodium or whether the natriuretic factor(s) had an effect on distal sodium transport as well. These data, nevertheless, indicate that the major site of natriuretic activity resides in the proximal tubule and there was a net loss of sodium. In RSW the increase in FEurate, an anion that is exclusively transported in the proximal tubule, supports our proposal that the major site of solute transport abnormality in RSW is in the proximal tubule and introduces the possibility that the natriuretic factor(s) might affect more than one transporter. (Maesaka & Fishbane, 1998) Moreover, these data do not have any similarities to the effects of A/BNP.

More recently, ammonium precipitates of urinary proteins of 5 of 6 neurosurgical patients with increased FEurate and normonatremia inhibited transcellular ^{22}Na transport in a dose-dependent manner across cultured pig proximal tubule cells, LLC-PK1, in transwells, as compared to precipitates from urine of neurosurgical patients with normal FEurate and normonatremia, and SIADH. (Youmans & Maesaka, 2011) These data support our previous studies in neurosurgical and AD, who had increased FEurate with normonatremia, an association that is highly suggestive of RSW. This conclusion is consistent with the frequency with which RSW is seen in neurosurgical diseases, with and without hyponatremia, see below. (Nelson et al, 1981; Sivakumar et al, 1994; Singh et al, 2002; Wijdicks et al, 1985)

3. Controversy over the relative prevalence of RSW and SIADH

The consistent view among internists and nephrologists is that RSW is a rare entity as compared to neurosurgeons, who consider RSW to be a common disorder. This important controversy exists because of the difficulty with which one syndrome can be differentiated from the other by usual clinical criteria. Because of overlapping clinical parameters such as hyponatremia, concentrated urines with high UNa, hypouricemia, increased FEurate, associations with intracranial diseases and normal renal, thyroid and adrenal function, there is a diagnostic dilemma that must be resolved in order to arrive at an appropriate therapeutic strategy for both syndromes. The only difference on first exposure with the patient is the volume depletion in RSW and increased volume in SIADH. (Bitew et al, 2009; Schwartz et al, 1957) Unfortunately, the clinical assessment of the volume status of non-edematous patients has been regarded as consistently inaccurate by usual clinical criteria. (Chung et al, 1987; Maesaka et al, 1999; Oh & Carroll; 1999; Singh et al, 2002)

We and others have encountered patients with RSW, who became symptomatic while being water-restricted for an erroneous diagnosis of SIADH. (Gutierrez et al ,2007; Maesaka et al, 1990,2007; Wijdicks et al, 1985) The common teaching that RSW is a rare clinical entity virtually eliminates its consideration when encountering patients with nonedematous hyponatremia. Because the major diagnostic conundrum rests with the volume status of these patients, we will review volume studies, mainly in neurosurgical patients, and offer strategies by which we can differentiate one syndrome from the other. In our view, the myriad of studies that have been published on cerebral/renal salt wasting, including the original report on cerebral salt wasting, has not adequately supported the diagnosis of RSW and have contributed to misconceptions. We will attempt to identify parameters by which the diagnosis of RSW can be made in order of their priority. We hope this review will provide information that will allow the reader to assess critically the merit of manuscripts on RSW and SIADH.

4. Evolution of the controversy over the existence and prevalence of RSW

The derivation of the controversy regarding the existence and relative prevalence of RSW and SIADH can be appreciated by a brief review of salt balance in normal subjects. Studies in Yanomamo Indians, the "no salt society", support the notion that we require virtually no salt in our diet to maintain normal ECV. (Hollenberg, 1980; Oliver et al, 1975) In Yanomamo Indians, the mean sodium excretion is 1 mmol/day, mean serum sodium 140 mmol/L, mean urine volume 1 L/day and mean blood pressure 102/62 mmHg. (Oliver et al, 1975) These studies suggest that we require little or no salt in our diets to maintain normal ECV.

Normal kidneys appear to have an innate sense of what is a normal ECV for that individual and adjust to any fluctuations in sodium intake to maintain ECV within narrow limits. (Hollenberg, 1980) The adjustments, however, are not instantaneous as sodium excretion will exceed input for up to 5 days before reaching equilibrium after an acute reduction in sodium intake. (Valtin, 1997) When a normal subject is placed in negative sodium balance by increasing urinary sodium excretion by diuretics or increased sweating, urinary sodium excretion decreases to as low as 1 mmol/day. (McCance, 1936; Strauss et al, 1958) Sodium excretion does not increase until the sodium losses have been replenished. (McCance, 1936; Strauss et al, 1958) This important role of normal kidneys to conserve sodium, when in a state of negative sodium balance is, in retrospect, the basis for the birth of the term cerebral salt wasting syndrome in 1950. (Peters et al, 1950) Peters et al reported 3 subjects with cerebral disease, acute encephalitis, subarachnoid hemorrhage and bulbar poliomyelitis. They concluded unconvincingly that these patients presented evidence of salt wasting, which was characterized by nitrogen retention, low blood pressure and correction of their hyponatremia by large salt intake. Nitrogen retention occurs in a volume depleted patient, referred to as prerenal azotemia, with retention of urea or nonprotein nitrogen (NPN), approximately double the BUN. (Abuelo, 2007) This is a reasonable assumption because urea excretion increases with any increase in urine output, even in RSW during volume repletion. (Shannon, 1936) NPN decreased from a baseline 44 to 25 mg/dL after receiving large amounts of salt in the first case. Only one NPN determination was reported in the second case with SAH and none was reported in the third case with bulbar poliomyelitis. The blood pressure in the first patient was 110/70 mmHg when the NPN was 44 mg/dL with preceding blood pressures of 120/80 to 130/88 mmHg without testing for postural changes in blood pressure or pulse. The second patient with SAH had one blood pressure reading of 220/110 mmHg and none was reported for the third case. The hyponatremia in all 3 patients did not respond to long periods of increased salt intake. The salt balance study that lasted 39 hours revealed the patient to be in negative sodium balance after salt intake was acutely reduced from 15 g/day to no salt intake. This delay in reaching equilibrium on the third day after an acute reduction in salt intake was construed as salt wasting, but is actually consistent with observations made in normal subjects. (Valtin, 1997) The negative sodium balance for 39 hours after an acute reduction in sodium intake does not justify the diagnosis of salt wasting. The first "dehydrated"case, however, could have had salt wasting. McCance and Strauss et al reported that a volume depleted subjects would avidly conserve sodium until their sodium losses were replaced. (McCance, 1936; Strauss et al, 1958) This "dehydrated" or assumed volume depleted patient had a urine chloride of 61.6 mmol/L, which can be explained by RSW. The inability to assess clinically the state of ECV has been the basis for doubting the existence of RSW. The same shortcomings were repeated in another report by the same authors on salt wasting. (Welt et al, 1952)

Four years later, Cort reported a hyponatremic patient with astrocytoma and papilledema, who had signs of dehydration. (Cort, 1954) Sodium intake of 15 g/day for many days failed to correct the hyponatremia. In a nine-day balance study, sodium intake was acutely reduced to 142.5 mg/day. The patient received corticotrophin on days 4, 5 and 6, deoxycorone on days 7, 8 and 9 and restarted on 15 mg/day salt on day 10. The patient went into negative sodium balance of 100 mmol on the first day and 60-70 mmol/day for the next 8 days. Sodium balance was unaffected by corticotrophin or deoxycortone. This study was compared to a similar study by McCance, who found normal subjects to go into sodium balance by the 5th day. (Cort, 1954) Determinations of daily chloride space revealed a 1.4 L reduction on the first day and 690 ml on the 9th day. Resumption of 15 g/day salt intake increased the chloride space by 1 L and her serum sodium "restored toward normal". (Cort, 1954) The reduction in chloride space and prolonged negative sodium balance prove the existence of RSW.

In 1957 Schwartz et al published their seminal report on SIADH that captured the fancy of physiologists and clinicians by reproducing the data in studies of vasopressin injections in healthy subjects by Leaf et al to propose the inappropriate secretion of ADH without the benefit of measuring plasma ADH levels. (Leaf et al, 1953; Schwartz et al, 1957) They proved convincingly that a hyponatremic patient, who presents with a concentrated urine, high UNa and increased ECV, as determined by radiosulfate measurements of ECV, must be due to an inappropriate secretion of ADH. ADH did not respond to the usual volume or osmolar stimuli and thus termed it inappropriate. The hyponatremia that was associated with a high UNa of 70 mmol/L and euvolemia or hypervolemia strengthened by determination of radiosulfate space, defined a syndrome that was not consistent with cerebral or renal salt wasting. (Schwartz et al, 1957)

There are several characteristics of SIADH that are worth reviewing as they relate to hyponatremia. These patients go into a period of negative sodium balance followed by an equilibrated state when sodium intake matches output. (Janenike & Waterhouse,1961) There is an increased blood volume as determined by sulfate space and by radioiodinated serum albumin and ^{51}Cr labeled red blood cells. (Bitew et al, 2009; Schwartz et al, 1957) The hypervolemia reduces plasma renin and aldosterone and increase plasma A/BNP. (Bitew et al, 2009; Fichman et al, 1974) GFR increases and urine osmolality is invariably concentrated. (Beck, 1979) Urine osmolality can, however, be dilute under circumstances of "ADH escape". Dilute urines have been noted after rapid infusion of saline at 2 L over a 2 hr period and after reducing sodium intake. (Jaenike & Waterhouse, 1961; Schwartz et al, 1957) Several possible explanations for this interesting phenomenon include a down regulation of V_2 receptor or increased urine flow rates cannot equilibrate with the hypertonic medulla. (Hoorn et al, 2005)

An unappreciated observation is an increase in serum sodium despite high fluid intake in SIADH. A balance study reported an increase in serum sodium from 105 to 135mmol/L over an 8 day period, when the mean fluid intake was 2648 ml/day and mean daily sodium intake of 315 mmol/day. The mean sodium concentration of 124.4 mmol/L in the input fluid was higher than the mean UNa of 86.8 mmol/l over the 8 day period. The sodium concentration in the intake fluid exceeded UNa on every day of the study, suggesting that serum sodium can increase even in SIADH as long as sodium concentration in the intake fluid exceeds UNa, regardless of the intake volume. (Schwartz et al, 1957) This reasoning can be applied to desalination when saline infusion decreases serum sodium. (Steele et al,1997). In the first case of SIADH, serum sodium decreased from 121 to 114 mmol/L after saline infusion when UNa was 70 mmol/L and to 103 mmol/L after hypertonic saline before undergoing a metabolic study. It is unlikely that serum sodium decreased while receiving saline, with a sodium concentration of 155 mmol/L, when UNa was 70 mmol/L. This is not consistent with desalination. (Steele et al, 1997) The best explanation for this phenomenon is an unrecorded intake of water that decreased the input sodium concentration below UNa. (Schwartz et al, 1957)

These elegantly designed studies in the initial report of SIADH proved that a hyponatremic patient can have high UNa without invoking RSW, largely because the volume status was shown to be increased by credible methods of determining ECV and not by tenuous clinical criteria as in the original report. (Peters et al, 1950) The existence of cerebral salt wasting was appropriately questioned. Since the assessment of ECV is critical in differentiating SIADH from RSW, it would be appropriate to review the various methods by which we assess ECV.

5. Assessment of extracellular volume

It is generally agreed that the assessment of ECV by clinical criteria is fraught with inaccuracies that the term "appeared dehydrated" is not acceptable for clinical and research purposes. (Chung et al, 1987; Maesaka et al, 1999; Oh & Carroll, 1999; Singh et al, 2002) The usual criteria of tissue turgor, axillary sweat, dry mucus membranes, neck vein distention or even postural hypotension in a nonedematous patient have been collectively inaccurate in assessing ECV. Even the presence of postural hypotension must consider autonomic dysfunction as we reported in a hyponatremic patient with autonomic failure and SIADH, proven by increased blood volume by gold standard radioisotope-dilution methods and depressed plasma renin and aldosterone. (Bitew et al, 2009) The use of plasma renin and aldosterone to differentiate SIADH from RSW can be helpful under ideal circumstances. In SIADH, plasma renin and aldosterone levels should be depressed, reflecting a slightly hypervolemic state, while in RSW, both levels should be increased, reflecting volume depletion. Clinically, however, determinations of plasma renin and aldosterone are delayed. Their diagnostic value is limited by a variety of exogenous factors. They include medication like ACE inhibitors, ARBs, B-Blockers, NSAIDS, heparin, diuretics and hyperuricemia. (Mulatero et al, 2002; Eraranta et al, 2008) A/BNP has not been used to differentiate SIADH from RSW.

It appears that noninvasive methods to assess ECV have limited value. Invasive methods have also been limited by various factors. A commonly used parameter is to measure central venous pressures (CVP). CVP has a poor correlation with concomitant radioisotope dilution measurements of blood volume and is also being discarded as a guide to fluid management. (Marik et al, 2008) The use of bioimpedance to determine volume in different compartments of the body is not useful as a single determination. (Schneditz, 2006)) Pulmonary wedge pressures are limited by a failure consistently to predict ECV but also by their invasiveness. (Godje et al, 1998)

There are two credible methods that can reliably determine ECV with greater accuracy than methods discussed above. One is the gold standard radioisotope-dilution method, using radioiodinated serum albumin and/or ^{51}Cr-tagged red blood cells, and the other, determination of total body water by deuterium and extracellular water by sodium bromide. As will be discussed below, there are a limited number of studies using radioisotope-dilution methods in SIADH and RSW and none using measurements of total and extracellular water in either of these two groups of patients.

5.1 Volume studies using radioisotope-dilution and other pertinent methodologies

As reviewed above, estimates of ECV have been made by determining chloride and thiosulfate spaces to support other criteria to establish the diagnosis of RSW and SIADH, respectively. (Cort, 1954; Schwartz et al, 1957) The gold standard for determining blood volume is by radioisotope dilution methods including radioiodinated serum albumin and/or ^{51}Cr labeled red blood cells. A study of 12 neurosurgical hyponatremic patients with UNa ranging from 41-203 mmol/L had blood volume determined by ^{51}Cr tagged red cells and radioiodinated serum albumin. Ten of the 12 patients had decreased blood volume and 2 had increased blood volume as compared to 6 control patients. (Nelson et al, 1981) The high UNa of 41 to 203 mmol/L suggests that 83.3% had RSW and 16.7% had SIADH. Eight patients had subarachnoid hemorrhage (SAH). In another study, plasma volume was determined by radioiodinated serum albumin in 21 patients on the first day of admission within 48 hours after SAH and on the 6th day after SAH. Comparisons between the first and second volume determination revealed blood volume to decrease in 8 of 9 hyponatremic patients, suggesting that 88.9% had RSW and 11.1% had SIADH. UNa values were not reported. (Wijdicks et al, 1985) Interestingly, plasma volume was decreased in 8, 66.7%, and increased in 4, 33.3%, of 12 nonhyponatremic patients with SAH, suggesting that RSW can occur in nonhyponatremic patients. Moreover, all 8 hyponatremic and 8 of 12 nonhyponatremic patients with decreased blood volume were in negative sodium balance. The increased blood volume in the 4 patients with normonatremia raises the question of whether or not SIADH can occur with normonatremia. In a separate study, Water restriction in volume depleted patients with SAH increased morbidity and mortality, probably due to decreased perfusion of brain and extension of ischemia in an already compromised circulation. (Wijdicks et al, 1985)

Another study used ^{51}Cr tagged red cells and CVP measurements in 18 hyponatremic patients of various etiologies with UNa of 43-210 mmol/L. (Sivakumar et al, 1994) Seventeen of 18 patients had decreased blood volumes, 18 of 18 patients had decreased CVP and all 18 patients corrected their hyponatremia within 72 hours after initiating saline infusion. The high UNa, decreased blood volume and correction of hyponatremia within 72 hours after initiating saline therapy argue strongly for RSW. We demonstrated a similar correction of hyponatremia within 48 hours after initiation of saline therapy in two patients with RSW and failure of saline therapy to correct the hyponatremia in two patients with SIADH. (Bitew et al, 2009; Maesaka et al, 2007) The three neurosurgical studies demonstrate by acceptable methods of determining ECV, that RSW is much more common than SIADH in neurosurgical patients, especially SAH.

A study in neurosurgical patients determined blood volume by ^{51}Cr labeled red cells in 20 hyponatremic and 20 nonhyponatremic "control" patients. Patients with evidence of "dehydration or hypovolemia" were excluded. All met criteria for SIADH. (Brimioulle et al, 2008) The exclusion of dehydrated or hypovolemic patients might have excluded patients with RSW and meeting the criteria for SIADH would include patients with RSW. Blood volumes were found to be comparable in the "control" and hyponatremic groups, suggesting that the hyponatremic group was entirely SIADH. Interestingly both the "control" and experimental groups were hypouricemic, mean serum urate 2.7 and 1.3 mg/dL and had high mean FEurate of 19% and 32% (normal 5-10%), respectively. There is ample evidence to suggest that the high FEurate in the hyponatremic group was consistent with both SIADH and RSW, while the nonhyponatremic group with increased FEurate would be consistent with RSW or normal controls depending on whether the FEurate was high or normal, respectively, figures 3, 4, table 1. (Maesaka et al, 1996, 1998, 1999, 2009) Based on these diagnostic possibilities, this study suffers first from a protocol-based elimination of patients with evidence of volume depletion as in RSW and failure to select the proper "control" and hyponatremic groups.

Ten patients with acquired immune deficiency syndrome with saline-responsive postural hypotension had CVP of 0 cm water, increased renin and aldosterone, hyponatremia, hypouricemia, elevated FEurate and UNa >40 mmol/l, which collectively support the diagnosis of RSW. (Cusano et al, 1990; Maesaka et al, 1990)

5.2 Other pertinent studies

In a retrospective study of 319 patients with SAH, 179 were hyponatremic and met criteria for SIADH and CSW. They found that 69.2% had SIADH, 6.5% CSW and 4.8% a combination of SIADH and CSW. The volume status was determined by CVP measurements, presence of hypotension and undefined parameters. This report suffers by its retrospective design, paucity of data to support their diagnoses and reliance on CVP measurements that have little value in assessing ECV. (Sherlock et al, 2006) In a similar retrospective study that included a variety of intracranial diseases, they found 62% of patients to have SIADH, 26.7% hypovolemic, 16.6% drug-related, 4.8% CSW, 3.7% related to IV fluids and 2.7% a combination of CSW and SIADH. In both studies, the combination of SIADH and CSW in 4.8% and 2.7% of patients lacked supportive data to justify such a difficult and improbable diagnostic combination, especially in a retrospective study. (Sherlock et al, 2006, 2009)

6. Renal salt wasting without clinical evidence of cerebral disease

To add further confusion to the dilemma of differentiating SIADH from RSW, we recently published 2 cases of unequivocal RSW without cerebral disease. (Bitew et al, 2009; Maesaka et al, 2007) One very instructive case was a hyponatremic patient with a hip fracture, who was initially water-restricted for 7 days for an erroneous diagnosis of SIADH by an internist. While being water-restricted, her Uosm was 362 mosm/kg and UNa only 6 mmol/L, which was initially construed as being consistent with hypovolemic hyponatremia of the prerenal type when UNa is typically low. A serum urate of 3.4 mg/dL, however, was not consistent with prerenal azotemia and more consistent with SIADH and RSW. A volume-depleted patient with normal kidney function would have higher serum urate with a FEurate below 3%. (Steele, 1969) Based on this reasoning, we performed a blood volume determination by gold standard radioisotope dilution methods and started saline infusion after baseline studies were collected. As expected the FEurate was markedly elevated at 29.6%, which was consistent with both SIADH and RSW, but a 7.1% reduction in blood volume was consistent with RSW. Increased baseline plasma renin and aldosterone and low normal ANP strongly supported the diagnosis of RSW. The low UNa of 6 mmol/L was attributed to a loss of appetite and reduced salt intake while being fluid-restricted to 750 ml/day for 7 days prior to our studies. She was feeling weak and anorectic while being fluid-restricted and felt stronger with increased appetite approximately 18 hours after initiating saline infusion. The baseline Uosm of 362 mosm/kg was attributed to a low medullary solute concentration resulting from low salt intake. A Uosm of 587 mosm/kg in the first urine passed after initiation of saline infusion supports our contention that the low salt intake decreased medullary solute concentration and decreased concentrating ability of the kidney, figure 1. The UNa of 6 mmol/L reflects her low sodium intake and reduction of renal medullary solute content. Moreover, saline infusion progressively diluted the urine to a Uosm of 152 mosm/kg 13 hours after initiating saline therapy, at which time plasma ADH decreased from a baseline of 1.9 pg/mL to indeterminate levels. The elimination of the volume stimulus for ADH production by saline allowed the coexisting hypo-osmolality to inhibit ADH production and induce excretion of dilute urines as serum sodium increased from a baseline 120 to 138 mmol/L in the next 48 hours, figure 1. (Maesaka et al, 2007)

Interestingly, the baseline FEurate of 29.6% increased further to a peak of 63% and 48% at the time of correction of the hyponatremia at 138 mmol/L, figure 2. The effect of saline on FEurate has been amply shown to be minimal. This persistently increased FEurate after correction of hyponatremia is consistent with RSW and not SIADH, to be discussed later. (Maesaka et al, 2007).

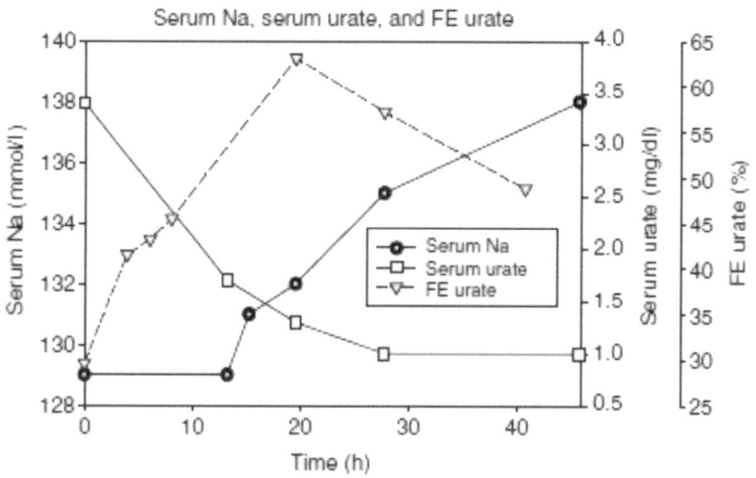

Fig. 2. Relationship between serum urate, serum sodium and FEurate during volume repletion with saline for 48 hours. Note that persistence of increased FEurate after correction of hyponatremia contrasts this to SIADH. Saline has been amply shown to have a meager effect on FEurate. (reproduced with permission from publisher)

In our view, this very instructive case followed predicted physiologic parameters for RSW and proved unequivocally the existence of RSW by collectively demonstrating the critical decrease in blood volume, increased plasma renin and aldosterone, low normal plasma ANP, appropriately increased plasma ADH, which was inhibited by the combination of volume repletion and hypo-osmolality, increased free water excretion, and timely correction of hyponatremia. These compelling data proved that RSW can occur without evidence of clinical cerebral disease and that a low sodium intake will be associated with a low UNa in a patient with RSW. (Maesaka et al, 2007)

7. Emerging value of determining FEurate

Determination of serum urate in SIADH was first reported in 1971. Patients with SIADH had hypouricemia and increased FEurate, which normalized after correction of the hyponatremia. (Dorhout Mees et al, 1971) In 1979 Beck duplicated these findings, but compared serum urate in SIADH with other causes of hyponatremia. Except for only one overlapping value, there was complete separation of serum urate in SIADH from other causes of hyponatremia. (Beck, 1979) Correcting the hyponatremia by water restriction was accompanied by an increase in serum urate with normalization of a previously increased FEurate, figures 3, 4. (Beck, 1979) Beck concluded that the coexistence of hyponatremia and hypouricemia differentiated SIADH from most other causes of hyponatremia. This apparent simple method of differentiating SIADH from other causes of hyponatremia stimulated others to investigate this relationship and renal urate handling. Serum urate was consistently found to be decreased in SIADH and there was virtually no overlap or partial overlap with other causes of hyponatremia. (Assadi & John, 1985; Passamonte 1984; Sonnenblick et al, 1988; Sorensen et al, 1988). FEurate was similarly increased in SIADH. (Assadi, 1985; Beck, 1979; Bitew, 2009; Decaux, 1990; Dorhout Mees ,1971; Drakakis, 2011; Weinberger et al, 1982; Sonnenblick, 1988; Sorenson, 1988) Several studies also demonstrated normalization or reduction of a previously increased FEurate after correction of hyponatremia by water restriction, figure 3, 4. (Assadi & John, 1985; Beck, 1979; Decaux et al, 1990; DorhoutMees et al, 1971; Drakakis et al, 2011; Sonnenblick et al, 1988) Improvements in hypouricemia and increased FEurate after correction of hyponatremia, appear to be characteristic findings in SIADH, but the coexistence of hypouricemia and hyponatremia has not been found as useful as FEurate, figures 3, 4.

We encountered 5 patients, in whom an increased FEurate and hypouricemia persisted after correction of their hyponatremia by water-restriction, suggesting that these hyponatremic patients were pathophysiologically different from SIADH. (Maesaka et al, 1990) The first patient had metastatic pancreatic carcinoma with hypoalbuminemia, albumin 1.5 g/dL, edema, ascites, hypouricemia (serum urate 1.1 mg/dL), increased FEurate, 34.2%, hypophosphatemia, 1.7 mg/dL, with increased FEphosphate, 29.1%, UNa 99mmol/L and Uosm 716 mosm/kg. His FEurate remained persistently increased at 30.0% after correction of hyponatremia to 138 mmol/L by water-restriction. The edema, ascites and increased FEphosphate were inconsistent with SIADH and the collective findings were consistent with a variant of the Fanconi syndrome. The second case was a patient with bronchogenic carcinoma with a negative CT scan of brain, who presented with serum sodium of 116 mmol/L, saline-responsive postural hypotension, Uosm 323 mosm/kg, UNa 42 mmol/L, serum urate 2.0 mg/dL, FEurate 26.5% and normal renal, adrenal and thyroid function. A diagnosis of SIADH was made on the basis of the report by Beck and he was water-restricted with liberal salt supplementation, which was followed by significant weight loss, recurrence of his postural hypotension, weakness, postural dizziness, slurred speech, staggered gait and somnolence. His serum sodium finally corrected to 138 mmol/l, and FEurate remained elevated at 14.7%, despite being severely volume depleted. At this time, his Uosm was 980 mosm/kg, UNa 181 mmol/L and he remained hypouricemic, serum urate 2.2 mg/dL. He responded well to saline therapy with reversal of all of his symptoms. The increased FEurate and hypouricemia persisted after correction of his hyponatremia by water restriction and salt supplementation, suggesting that a persistently elevated FEurate and hypouricemia after correction of hyponatremia would be consistent with RSW. We found a persistent increase in FEurate and hypouricemia after correction of hyponatremia in three additional cases, one with bronchogenic carcinoma that had metastasized to brain, another with disseminated Cryptococcus that involved brain and uncomplicated Hodgkins disease with no clinical cerebral disease. All had normal renal adrenal and thyroid function. The hyponatremia, high UNa and concentrated urine were consistent with SIADH except for the persistent increase in FEurate. The hyponatremia, high UNa and concentrated urine were consistent with SIADH except for the persistent increase in FEurate, which was construed as being pathophysiologically different from SIADH and might serve to differentiate SIADH from RSW, figure 3, 4. Moreover, the absence of clinical cerebral disease in 3 of the 5 patients raised questions regarding the appropriateness of the term cerebral salt wasting.

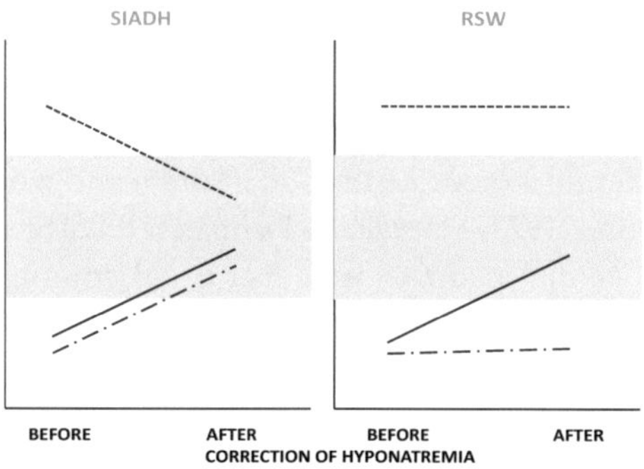

Fig. 3.

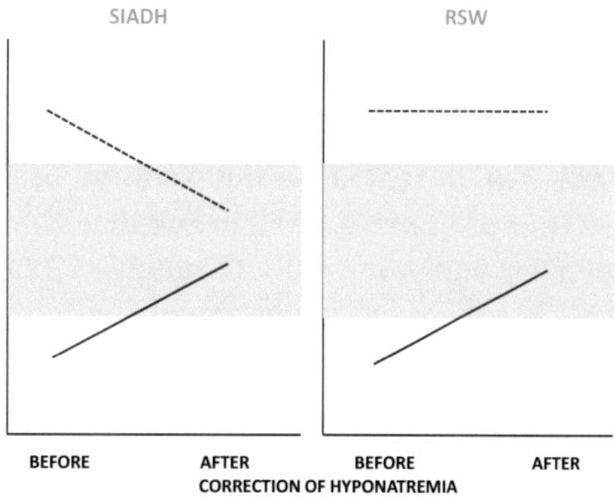

Fig. 4.

Fig. 3. and 4. Relationship between FEurate (FEUA ....), serum urate (SUA — . —) and serum sodium (SNa ———) before and after correction of hyponatremia in SIADH and RSW. Shaded areas represent normal ranges. (Modified from Maesaka, 1999), Figure 3. Figure 4 is updated version with elimination of SUA, see test.

We prospectively evaluated 96 patients with AIDS. Sixteen patients had combined hyponatremia and hypouricemia, 21 were hypouricemic, and 19 of 23 patients studied had increased FEurate. Many had increased FEurate with normonatremia, which was consistent with RSW and not SIADH. All hyponatremic patients had high UNa and concentrated urines that were consistent with SIADH and RSW. Ten hyponatremic patients with saline responsive postural hypotension, CVP of 0 cm H_2O with high plasma renin and aldosterone collectively supported a diagnosis of RSW in AIDS. (Maesaka et al, 1990, 1990)

We extended our study to neurosurgical patients with diverse etiologies because 12 of 12 hypouricemia patients with AIDS had cortical atrophy of brain by CT scan. (Maesaka et al, 1990, 1992) The high incidence of RSW in neurosurgical patients suggested that RSW in AIDS might be due to their cerebral disease, so we prospectively studied urate metabolism in 29 neurosurgical patients of varying etiologies and 21 age and gender-matched controls. Seven patients were hypouricemic, 18 had FEurate > 10% and only 1 patient was hyponatremic. (Maesaka et al, 1992) We postulated that the increase in FEurate without hyponatremia was again consistent with RSW that was supported by the volume studies in neurosurgical patients. These observations solidified our notion that an increased FEurate with normonatremia may be consistent with RSW without a need to correct hyponatremia, figures 3, 4. Moreover, an increased FEurate was associated with serum urate > 5 mg/dL, suggesting a greater value of FEurate over serum urate. (Maesaka et al, 1992, 1998, 2009)

A study of urate metabolism focused on other cerebral diseases because patients with AD were reported to have lower serum urate. (Kasa et al, 1989) Serum urate was lower and FEurate higher in 18 patients with AD as compared to 6 patients with multi infarct dementia and 11 age and gender-matched normal controls. (Maesaka et al, 1993) As in the neurosurgical study, only one patient with AD was hyponatremic. The increased FEurate with normonatremia suggested that demented patients with AD might have RSW and raised the question whether or not an isolated increase in FEurate with normonatremia without prior correction of a pre-existing hyponatremia would be consistent with RSW.

One drawback to our proposal of determining FEurate after correction of hyponatremia to differentiate SIADH from RSW was the unpredictability of correcting the hyponatremia. We utilized the recommendation to treat hyponatremic patients with cerebral disease with hypertonic saline, regardless of whether or not the patient had SIADH or RSW. (Sterns et al, 2008) We increased serum sodium to 138 mmol/L within 2-3 days with 1.5% and determined FEurate, being aware that saline had only a modest effect on FEurate and would not likely alter our results. (Cannon, 1970; Diamond, 1975; Maesaka & Fishbane, 1998; Steele, 1974) We corrected hyponatremia within 2-3 days in 3 patients, who met usual criteria for SIADH, and found a previously increased FEurate to decrease to < 10% in all 3 patients. (Drakakis et al, 2011) Normalization of FEurate after correction of hyponatremia can be predictably achieved in 2-3 days by hypertonic saline and can be contrasted to a persistent increase in FEurate in RSW, figures 3, 4. The rate of correction can be controlled by monitoring serum sodium and adjusting free water intake to achieve the desired rate and extent of the correction of hyponatremia. These studies confirmed our notion that saline has a meager effect on FEurate by decreasing to normal levels during saline infusion. Under the proper circumstances of adequate cardiac function, hyponatremia can be corrected with 1.5% hypertonic saline in a predictably timely fashion to differentiate SIADH from RSW, figures 3, 4. (Drakakis et al, 2011)

7.1 Pathophysiology of increased FEurate in SIADH and RSW

The mechanisms by which FEurate increases in both SIADH and RSW are presently unexplained. The most prominent explanation has been the volume expansion that is seen in SIADH, but the saline infusion studies suggest that volume expansion has only a meager effect on FEurate. (Cannon et al, 1970; Diamond et al, 1975; Steele et al, 197) The V_1 ADH receptor has been proposed as a cause for the increase in FEurate in SIADH after demonstrating an increase in FEurate by pitressin, and eliminating the effect by a V_1-specific receptor inhibitor. (Decaux et al, 1996) This explanation is untenable because FEurate increased significantly at a time when normal subjects were hyponatremic during intranasal dDAVP, which lacks V_1 activity, and by normalization of FEurate with correction of hyponatremia in SIADH when plasma ADH levels are still elevated. (Boer et al, 1987) It has been proposed that the defect in urate transport in SIADH was a result of an inhibition of the post secretory reabsorptive site for urate transport, based on the combination of the assumed secretory inhibition by pyrazinamide and decrease in post secretory reabsorption of urate by sulfapyrazone. (Weinberger et al, 1982) Studies in brush border membranes, however, demonstrate increased uptake of urate in the presence of pyrazinamide, suggesting that the decrease in urate excretion during pyrazinamide administration was a result of increased reabsorption and not inhibition of secretion. (Roch-Ramel et al, 1994) Until there is further clarification of the mechanisms and sites at which urate is transported, we must conclude that there is increased FEurate at a time when the patient is hyponatremic in SIADH, but the mechanism for this unique transport abnormality remains unclear. Lastly, the proposal that the chronic hyponatremia or hypo-osmolality contributed to the increase in FEurate in SIADH cannot be supported by the normal FEurate that has been reported in hyponatremia due to psychogenic polydipsia and more recently, RO, to be discussed below. (Ali et al, 2009; Decaux et al, 2000; Imbriano et al, 2011)

The increased FEurate in RSW, like that in SIADH, is presently not understood. There is a natriuretic factor(s) that is present in plasma and urine of patients with neurosurgical diseases and in plasma of patients with AD. As discussed above, this factor(s) has a major inhibitory effect on proximal tubule sodium transport. (Maesaka et al, 1993, 1993; Youmans & Maesaka, 2011) The proximal tubule is the exclusive site of urate reabsorption and predominant site for phosphate. It would be interesting to speculate that the natriuretic factor might have a dose-dependent effect with different affinities for various transporters in the proximal tubule. The circulating factor could also explain the persistent increase in FEurate after correction of hyponatremia in RSW. Consistent with this speculation is our patient with metastatic pancreatic cancer who had transport defects for sodium, urate and phosphate that were interpreted as being consistent with the Fanconi syndrome. (Maesaka et al, 1990) For the moment, however, there are few insights into mechanisms by which FEurate increases in RSW.

7.2 Hyponatremia with normal FEurate in reset osmostat

Further appreciation of the emerging importance of determining FEurate in hyponatremic patients comes from our study of patients with RO or type C SIADH, which accounts for 36% of patients with SIADH. (Zerbe et al, 1980) It is characterized by euvolemia with normal renal, adrenal and thyroid function, hyponatremia resulting from ADH stimulation at a lower plasma osmolality or a RO, having a reasonably normal diluting and concentrating capacity of urine, and maintaining normal sodium balance without correcting the hyponatremia. (Wall, 1993) They are typically untreated, but this approach poses a therapeutic dilemma because of our tendency to treat most if not all hyponatremics. (DeFronzo et al, 1976; Decaux et al, 2009; Elisaf et al, 1990; Hill et al, 1990; Kahn, 2003) We encountered 3 patients with hyponatremia and normal FEurate, who were noted to excrete urines with Uosm < 200 mosm/kg, that was consistent with RO. Based on these findings, we decided to perform water-loading tests in nonedematous hyponatremic patients with normal FEurates without a dilute urine in a randomly collected urine, regardless of UNa or serum urate. (Imbriano, 2011) In this study of 14 patients, every nonedematous hyponatremic patient we encountered with a FEurate of 4-10% had RO as determined by Uosm <200 mosm/kg on a random urine collection, 8 patients, or after a normal water-loading test, 6 patients. As is typical of RO, plasma ADH was undetectable in 4 patients studied during the water-loading test. Eleven patients had UNa > 20 mmol/L, 8 were hypouricemic, yet all had a normal FEurate of < 10%. Interestingly, 3 patients were on losartan and 2 on atorvastatin, which increase urine urate excretion and lower serum urate. (Milionis et al, 2004; Yamamoto et al, 2000) These data suggest that chronic hyponatremia does not increase FEurate as has been proposed as a contributing factor for the increased FEurate in SIADH. (Decaux et al 2000) Comorbid conditions were similar to those reported in RO, including 2 patients without comorbidities. These and our other studies refine the proposal by Beck, that the coexistence of hyponatremia and hypouricemia differentiates SIADH from most other causes of hyponatremia, by stressing the greater value of FEurate over serum urate. (Beck, 1979; Maesaka et al, 1998, 2009) We concluded that RO occurs commonly, a normal FEurate in a nonedematous hyponatremic patient is highly suggestive of RO and FEurate has greater clinical utility than serum urate. (Imbriano et al, 2011) FEurate has a physiological basis for its derivation as compared to multiple factors that determine serum urate, including endogenous or exogenous purine sources, endogenous production and excretion via gut and urine. Moreover, the arbitrary definition of hypouricemia ranging from 1.5-4 mg/dL reflect the uncertainty of the value of serum urate as compared to well-defined parameters that have been established for FEurate. (Beck, 1979; Maesaka et al, 1990 e; Ramsdell & Kelley, 1973) These studies also introduce the possibility that RO is pathophysiologically different from the more traditional SIADH by virtue of the normal FEurate and predictability of ADH responses to plasma osmolality.

8. Change cerebral salt wasting to renal salt wasting

The 2 cases of RSW without clinical cerebral disease were the impetus to propose replacing the designation, cerebral salt wasting, to renal salt wasting. (Bitew et al, 2009; Maesaka et al, 2007, 2009) Based on these reports, cerebral salt wasting should be considered an outmoded and inappropriate designation; it should now be called RSW because RSW will be considered in any hyponatremic patient with or without cerebral disease. (Maesaka et al, 2009) Although we feel that RSW might be rare in patients without clinical cerebral disease, these cases of RSW without clinical cerebral disease support our contention that the true prevalence of RSW cannot be viewed as rare until future studies can accurately determine the prevalence of SIADH and RSW in patients with and without clinical evidence of cerebral disease. This would depend on our ability to differentiate SIADH from RSW. The volume studies indicate that RSW is much more common than SIADH in neurosurgical patients. We hope this expanded approach to hyponatremia and RSW will eliminate the inappropriate treatment of RSW by fluid restriction, which has been shown to increase morbidity and mortality when misdiagnosed as SIADH. (, Gutierrez & Lin, 2009; Maesaka et al, 1990, 2007; Wijdicks et al, 1985)

9. New approach to hyponatremia and how to differentiate SIADH from RSW

The evaluation of the patient with hyponatremia traditionally starts with an assessment of ECV, whether or not they are euvolemic, hypovolemic or hypervolemic. While this approach is fundamentally correct, we are again unable to assess accurately whether the patient is euvolemic or hypovolemic, realizing that hypervolemic patients can be identified by the presence of edema. We attempted to use UNa to support the volume approach by dividing the hypovolemic group into two categories, those with hypovolemia and normal kidney function, UNa < 20 mmol/L and those with rSW, UNa > 20 mmol/L. Those with euvolemia or mainly SIADH, UNa is usually > 20 mmol/L and hypervolemia, UNa < 20 mmol/L. The major differential is a UNa of > 20 mmol/L, which reverts back to differentiating SIADH from RSW. Differentiating the hypovolemic patient with normal renal function from hypervolemic hyponatremics, UNa < 20 mmol/L, is simplified by the presence or absence of edema. (Maesaka, 1996) The interpretation of UNa is also complicated by many factors, such as diuretics, the acutely vomiting patient with bicarbonaturia, acute and chronic kidney diseases and low UNa in the patient with SIADH and RSW on a low sodium diet. Limitations of UNa in the evaluation of patients with hyponatremia have been noted by others. (Chung et al, 1987)

Determinations of plasma renin and aldosterone can under proper circumstances contribute to differentiating SIADH from RSW. However, many factors can affect one or both values, such as the use of diuretics, ACE inhibitors, ARB, NSAIDS, heparin or saline.(Mulatero et al,

2002) Even under ideal circumstances the delay in obtaining these results does not assist us on first encounter with the patient.

It is evident that the evaluation of the volume status or determining UNa has limited utility. This dilemma persists to this day on first encounter with the nonedematous hyponatremic patient. We developed an algorithm, which emphasizes FEurate in the evaluation of hyponatremia, table 1. We propose with supporting data to determine FEurate in any nonedematous patient with hyponatremia. If the FEurate is 5-10%, we should consider psychogenic polydipsia, RO and prerenal causes, such as congestive heart failure, cirrhosis, nephrosis and pre eclampsia, or hypovolemia with normal renal function. Psychogenic polydipsia can be eliminated from the history of increased water intake and very dilute urines. (Ali et al, 2009) Edematous states can be ruled out by the presence of edema. The major obstacle might be the hypovolemic patient with normal renal function and classic prerenal azotemia, but the low mean FEurate of 2.85%, possibly high serum urate and UNa < 20 mmol/l might assist in differentiating this group from RO. (Steele, 1969) In patients who do not fall into the groups mentioned, we would consider RO and search diligently for a dilute urine in a random urine collection. In the absence of a dilute random urine, we do not recommend performing a water-loading test to prove the diagnosis of RO. (Imbriano et al, 2011) We would instead treat them with water restriction and salt supplementation, however unsuccessful they are, and consider using ADH receptor inhibitors, vaptans.

If the FEurate exceeds preferably 12%, there are three possibilities to consider, SIADH, RSW, thiazide diuretics and drugs that induce an SIADH-like picture. Thiazide diuretics and neurotropics can be readily eliminated by a proper history so the major differential would be SIADH and RSW. We propose to correct serum sodium either by water-restriction with salt supplementation or 1.5% hypertonic saline and determine FEurate. (Drakakis et al, 2011) If FEurate corrects to < 10%, we would proceed with treatment for SIADH or if it exceeds 10%, preferably >12%, we would treat the patient for RSW with saline. The question represented as dotted lines in table 1 depends on whether the coexistence of increased FEurate with normonatremia would be diagnostic of RSW. While there are supporting data to suggest this to be a valid conclusion, especially in patients with neurosurgical diseases, future studies will hopefully provide further insights into this relationship. Because neurosurgical patients are routinely treated with hypertonic saline, an increased FEurate with normonatremia or hypernatremia would be suggestive of RSW, see above. We have found this algorithm to be superior to the previous approach as discussed above and expect to make further refinements to this algorithm in the future.

10. Treatment of the hyponatremic patient with SIADH and RSW

The increasing reports of significant symptoms being attributed to even mild hyponatremia not only shed light on a long unrecognized phenomenon, but introduce the need for some urgency in developing adequate treatment strategies for a condition with diverse etiologies and divergent therapeutic goals. Treatment, however, has undergone a period of uncertainty due to adverse outcomes that are related to delays in treatment and over-correction of chronic hyponatremia. (Berl et al, 1990) The approach to methods of correction in different clinical conditions will be limited to SIADH and RSW and the reader is referred to broader reviews of treating hyponatremia. (Stern et al, 2009; Verbalis et al, 2007) As discussed earlier, foremost among the diagnostic and therapeutic dilemma is the need to differentiate SIADH from RSW in order to fulfill divergent therapeutic goals. It is well known that severe hyponatremia can cause neurologic symptoms, such as irritability, seizures and even apnea, but more subtle alterations in memory and judgment, unsteady gait and even falls have been associated with mild hyponatremia that have responded to treatment of their hyponatremia. (Berl et al, 2010; Decaux et al, 2006, 2009; Gankam Kengne et al, 2008; Renneboog et al, 2006) It is, therefore, pertinent to ask whether "asymptomatic hyponatremia exists". (Schrier, 2010) One of the most alarming outcomes has been the descriptions of a four-fold increase in falls that have been attributed to mild hyponatremia, mean serum sodium 131 mmol/L, in the elderly. (Renneboog et al, 2006; Gankam Kengne et al, 2008) There is, therefore, a movement to consider treating all hyponatremics, including the infusion of hypertonic saline to treat hyponatremic patients with brain diseases to avoid brain edema regardless of whether or not they have SIADH or RSW. (Sterns & Silver, 2008)

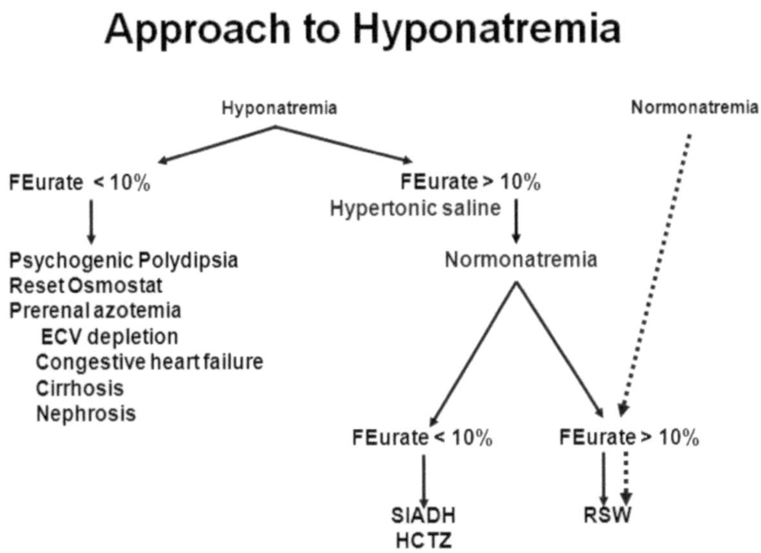

Table 1. New approach to hyponatremia based on FEurate. Normonatremia and FEurate without hyponatremia needs further verification, dotted line.

The standard approach to treating hyponatremia depends on the etiology of the hyponatremia. Patients with edematous causes of hyponatremia such as heart failure, cirrhosis or nephrosis are treated with a combination of water-restriction, low salt diet, diuretics and the ADH inhibitors or vaptans. Vaptans are clearly indicated in edematous states and are contraindicated in hypovolemic patients. Of the available vaptans, conivaptan inhibits the V_{1A} and V_2 receptor for ADH and tolvaptan the V_2 receptor. Conivaptan is administered only intravenously and inhibits CYP3A4 so its administration must consider other agents that might be metabolized by this pathway and potentially increase blood levels of conivaptan. (Sterns et al, 2009) Because conivaptan inhibits the V_{1A} receptor, which has vasopressive activity, it is not indicated for treatment of hyponatremic cirrhotics. (Sterns et al, 2009) SIADH and RO are treated by water-restriction with salt supplementation and hypertonic saline in patients with brain disease, but the vaptans appear to be promising for both conditions. Vaptans have been shown to increase serum sodium successfully and improve symptoms attributed to non hypovolemic hyponatremia, including better symptomatic improvement in patients with SIADH. (Berl et al, 2010; Schrier et al, 2006; Verbalis et al, 2011) Patients should not be water-restricted while being treated with the vaptans except under very unusual circumstances to avoid rapid correction of hyponatremia. Serum sodium should be monitored at least within 8 hours of initiating vaptan therapy, but we recommend repeating serum sodium determinations earlier if the patient increases urine output soon after starting vaptan therapy. (Berl et al, 2010) The increase in urine output suggests that ADH receptor inhibition is occurring rapidly and the resulting increase in free water excretion would correct sodium rapidly thereafter, hence a recommendation to determine serum sodium at this time. Over-correction of hyponatremia can be avoided by closely matching the increased urine volume or if too rapid, by the administration of free water and/or intranasal dDAVP.

The treatment of SIADH, including RO, traditionally starts with the treatment of the associated clinical condition, fluid restriction to < 1000 ml/day, salt supplementation, occasionally diuretics, demeclocyline and ADH inhibitors. The correction of hyponatremia in SIADH by fluid restriction and/or salt supplementation has been slow and often incomplete or unsuccessful. Treatment of RO has been generally unsuccessful to the point of not recommending any treatment for these patients. The use of vaptans in SIADH can be justified by their hypervolemic state, but it is uncertain whether patients with RO are similarly volume expanded. Although an increase in volume makes intuitive sense, volume studies have not been performed in patients with RO to justify use of vaptans . Our ability to identify patients with RO by virtue of a normal FEurate will uncover this common cause of hyponatremia and test the efficacy of vaptans in this therapeutically challenging group. (Imbriano et al, 2011)

In contrast to the difficulty of treating patients with SIADH or RO, the treatment of RSW is simple. Eliminating the appropriate volume stimulus for ADH secretion in this disorder with saline will allow the coexisting hypo-osmolality to inhibit ADH secretion, increase free water excretion and correct the hyponatremia. (Bitew et al, 2009; Maesaka et al, 2007) Use of vaptans is obviously contraindicated in these volume depleted patients. While the rationale for increasing salt and water intake in patients with RSW is obvious, we are again confronted with our inability to differentiate SIADH from RSW with any degree of certainty. This therapeutic dilemma has been partially resolved by the recommendation to treat hyponatremic patients with acute neurological/neurosurgical diseases with hypertonic saline to prevent the complications associated with brain edema of multiple causes. (Sterns & Silver, 2008 and et al, 2009) As discussed earlier, RSW is more common than SIADH in neurosurgical diseases and the use of hypertonic saline not only reduces brain edema but has other advantages, such as treating their volume depletion. (Sterns & Silver, 2008) Administration of hypertonic saline prevents hyponatremia from occurring so an increased FEurate would be consistent with RSW. (Youmans & Maesaka, 2011). A timely correction of an existing hyponatremia by judicious use of hypertonic saline can also differentiate SIADH from RSW, whether FEurate normalizes or remains increased, respectively, figures 3, 4.

Hyponatremic patients outside of the neurology/neurosurgical ICU, including those with nonedematous hyponatremia with or without cerebral disease, need to be evaluated for etiology of their hyponatremia, as discussed above. Following the algorithm in table 1 has been useful in our hands. Therapy will depend on the etiology of the hyponatremia. In those with increased FEurate, the diagnostic dilemma of differentiating SIADH from RSW must be extended to those without clinical cerebral disease. This diagnostic and dependent therapeutic dilemma will persist until we have a mindset to consider RSW in these patients and develop a better diagnostic approach to solving this dilemma. Recommendations to determine FEurate in normonatremic patients have not been resolved except to include it as a routine measurement in any patient with acute brain disease and demented patients with AD.

In patients with symptomatic hyponatremia such as muscular irritability, altered mental status or seizures, the patient should be treated with hypertonic saline to increase serum sodium by 4-6 mmol/l over 4 hours and then slowly thereafter. (Sterns & Silver, 2008) Although it is safe to increase serum sodium to normal values in conditions such as in acute and documented water intake, marathon runners, that cause acute hyponatremia, we recommend gradual improvement in all patients with hyponatremia to avoid any contributions rapid correction might add to circumstances in which osmotic demyelination might occur irrespective of their sodium, such as in malnourished patients or those with liver disease. (Almond et al, 2005, Sterns & Silver, 2008) We favor a conservative approach to the correction of chronic hyponatremia by increasing serum sodium <10 mmol/l/24 hrs with slower rates for patients with severe malnutrition and cirrhosis to avoid osmotic demyelination.

11. Summary

The present chapter hopefully provided the following important insights and new directions in our understanding of RSW:

1. an appreciation of the diagnostic and therapeutic dilemma that exists for SIADH and RSW.
2. provided an objective review of how the controversy over the relative prevalence of SIADH and RSW evolved.
3. emphasized our inability to assess accurately the state of ECV as being the root of this enigmatic controversy and how the overlapping features of both syndromes make it virtually impossible to differentiate SIADH from RSW on first encounter.
4. reviewed the relative merits by which we determine ECV.
5. RSW is much more common than SIADH in neurosurgical patients and RSW can occur in the absence of hyponatremia.
6. although FEurate is increased in both SIADH and RSW, FEurate can differentiate one syndrome from the other by reverting to normal in SIADH and being persistently increased after correction of hyponatremia.
7. the demonstration of natriuretic activity in plasma of neurosurgical and in the plasma and urine of Alzheimer disease patients with increased FEurate and normonatremia introduces the possibility that an increased FEurate with normonatremia might be diagnostic of RSW.
8. the natriuretic factor probably contributes to RSW, has its major effect in the proximal tubule where urate is exclusively transported and is not A/BNP.
9. a normal FEurate in patients with nonedematous hyponatremia is highly suggestive of RO and identifies a common and overlooked disorder.
10. the normal FEurate and predictability of ADH responses suggest that RO might represent a group that is pathophysiologically different from SIADH.

11. we provide a useful algorithm that utilizes FEurate as central to our approach to evaluating patients with hyponatremia.
12. based on our two cases of renal salt wasting without clinical cerebral disease, we propose eliminating the term cerebral salt wasting in favor of renal salt wasting

12. References

Abuelo JG: Normotensive ischemic acute renal failure. (2007) *N Eng Jour Med*,357,pp.797-8

Ali N, Imbriano L, Miyawaki N, & Maesaka JK.(2009) 66-year-old male with Hyponatremia. *Kidney Int*,76,pp.233-234

Almond CS, Shin AY, Fortescue EB, Mannix RC, Wypij D, Binstadt BA, Duncan CN, Olson DP, Salerno AE, Newburger JW, & Greenes DS. (2005) Hyponatremia among runners in the Boston Marathon. *N Engl J Me*,;352, pp.1550-1556

Arieff AI, Llach F, & Massry SG. (1976) Neurological manifestations and morbidity of hyponatremia: correlation with brain water and electrolytes. *Medicine (Baltimore)*,55(2),pp.121-129.

Assadi FK, & John EG. (11985) Hypouricemia in neonates with syndrome of inappropriate secretion of antidiuretic hormone. *Ped Res*,19,pp.424-427.

Beck LH. (1979) Hypouricemia in the syndrome of inappropriate secretion of antidiuretic hormone. *N Engl J Med*,301,pp.528-530

Berl T, Quittnat-Pelletier F, Verbalis JG, Schrier RW, Bichet DG, Ouyang J, & Czerwiec FS. (2010) SALTWATER Investigators. Oral tolvaptan is safe and effective in chronic hyponatremia. *J Am Soc Nephrol*,21(4),pp.705-712

Berl T, Quittnat-Pelletier F, Verbalis JG, Schrier RW, Bichet DG, Ouyang J, & Czerwiec FS; SALTWATER Investigators. (2010) Oral tolvaptan is safe and effective in chronic hyponatremia. *J Am Soc Nephrol*, 21,pp.705-712

Berl T. (1990) Treating hyponatremia: damned if we do and damned if we don't. Kidney Int. 37(3),pp.1006-1018.

Bitew S, Imbriano L, Miyawaki N, Fishbane S, & Maesaka JK. (2009) More on renal salt wasting without cerebral disease, response to saline infusion. *Clin J Amer Soc Nephol*,4:309-315

Boer WH, Koomans HA, & Dorhout Mees EJ. (1987) Lithium clearance during the paradoxical natriuresis of hypotonic expansion in man. *Kidney In*, 32,pp.376-381

Brimioulle S, Oretiani-Jimenez C, Aminian A, & Vincent JL.(2008) Hyponatremia in neurological patients: cerebral salt wasting versus inappropriate antidiuretic hormone secretion. *Intensive Care Med*,34,pp.125-131

Burnett JC Jr, Kao PC, Hu DC, Heser DW, Heublein D, Granger JP, Opgenorth TJ, & Reeder GS. (1986) Atrial natriuretic peptide elevation in congestive heart failure in the human. *Science*,7;231(4742),pp.1145-1147.

Cannon PJ, Svahn DS, & Demartini FE: (1970) The influence of hypertonic saline infusions upon the fractional reabsorption of urate and other ions in normal and hypertensive man. *Circulation*,41,pp.97-108..

Chung HM, Kluge R, Schrier RW, & Anderson RJ. (1987) Clinical assessment of extracellular fluid volume in hyponatremia. *Am J Med*,83,pp.905-908

Cort JH. (1954) Cerebral salt wasting. *Lancet*(1),pp.752-754

Cusano AJ, Thies HL, Siegal FP, Dreisbach AW, & Maesaka JK (1990) Hyponatremia in patients with acquired immunodeficiency syndrome. *Jour AIDS*,3,pp.949-953 de Zeeuw D, Janssen WM, & de Jong PE. (1992) Atrial natruretic factor: its (patho) physiological significance in humans. *Kidney Int*,41,pp. 1115-1133

Decaux G, Namias B, Gulbis B, & Soupart A: (1996) Evidence in hyponatremia related to inappropriate secretion of ADH that V1 receptor stimulation contributes to the increase in renal uric acid clearance. *J Am Soc Nephrol*,7,pp. 805-810.

Decaux G, Prospert F, Soupart A, & Musch W. (2000) Evidence that chronicity of hyponatremia contributes to the high urate clearance observed in the syndrome of inappropriate secretion of antidiuretic hormone. *Am J Kidney Dis* 36,pp.745-751

Decaux G. (2006) Is asymptomatic hyponatremia really asymptomatic? *Am J Med*,119 (7 Suppl 1),pp.S79-S82.

Decaux G. (2009) The syndrome of inappropriate secretion of antidiuretic hormone (SIADH). *Semin Nephrol*,29,pp.239-256.

DeFronzo RA, Goldberg M, & Agus Z. (1976) Normal diluting capacity in hyponatremic patients. Reset Osmostat or a variant of the syndrome of inappropriate hormone secretion. *Ann Int Med*, 84,pp.538-542

Diamond H, & Meisel A. (1975) Influence of volume expansion, serum sodium, and fractional excretion of sodium on urate excretion. *Pflugers Arch*,356,pp.47-57.

Dorhout Mees EJ, Blom van Assendelft P, & Nieuwenhuis MG: (1971) Elevation of urate clearance caused by inappropriate antidiuretic hormone secretion. *Acta Med*,189,pp.69-72

Dorhout Mees EJ. (1990) History of the "lithium concept". Kidney Int Suppl,28,pp.S2-S3.

Drakakis J, Imbriano L, Miyawaki N, Shirazian S, & Maesaka. (2011) Normalization of fractional excretion of urate (FEurate) after correction of hyponatremia differentiates SIADH from cerebral/renal salt wasting (RSW). Abst. *Annual Mtg Am Soc Nephrol*, Philadelphia, PA, USA

Elisaf MS, Konstantinides A, & Stamopoulos KC. (1996) Chronic hyponatremia due to reset osmostat in a patient with colon cancer. *Am J Nephrol*,16,pp.349-351.

Ellison DH, & Berl T. (2007) The syndrome of inappropriate antidiuresis. *N Engl J Med*,356,pp.2064-207

Eräranta A, Kurra V, Tahvanainen AM, Vehmas TI, Kööbi P, Lakkisto P, Tikkanen I, Niemelä OJ, Mustonen JT, & Pörsti IH. (2008) Oxonic acid-induced hyperuricemia elevates plasma aldosterone in experimental renal insufficiency. *J Hypertens*,26(8),pp.1661-8.

Fenske W, Stork S, Koschker AC, Blechschmidt A, Lorenz D, Wortmann S, & Allolio B. (2008)Value of fractional uric acid excretin in differential diagnosis of hyponatremic patients on diuretics. *J. Clin Endocrinol Metab*,93,pp.2991-2997

Fichman MP, Micheldakis AP, & Horton R. (1974) Regulation of aldosterone in the syndrome of inappropriate antidiuretic hormone secretion (SIADH): *J Clin Endocrinol Metab*,39,pp.136-144

Gankam Kengne F, Andres C, Sattar L, Melot C, & Decaux G. (2008) Mild hyponatremia and risk of fracture in the ambulatory elderly. *QJM*,101(7),pp.583-588.

Gödje O, Peyerl M, Seebauer T, Lamm P, Mair H, & Reichart B. (1998) Central venous pressure, pulmonary capillary wedge pressure and intrathoracic blood volumes as preload indicators in cardiac surgery patients. *Eur J Cardiothorac Surg*,13(5),pp.533-539

Gutierrez OM, & Lin HY: (2007) Refractory Hyponatremia. *Kidney Int*,71,pp.79-82

Hill RA, Uribarri J, Mann J, & Berl T. (1990) Altered water metabolism in tuberculosis: role of vasopressin. *Am J Med*,88,pp.357-364.

Hollenberg NK. (1980) Set point for sodium homeostasis: Surfeit, deficit, and their implication. *Kidney Int*,17,pp.423-429.

Hoorn EJ, Hoffert JD, & Knepper MA. (2005) Combined proteomics and pathways analysis of collecting duct reveals a protein regulatory network activated in vasopressin escape. *J Am oc Nephrol*, 16, pp.2852-2863

Hoorn EJ, Van Der Lubbe N, Zietse R. (2009) SIADH and hyponatremia: why does it matter. NDT plus (suppl 3),pp. iii5-iii11

Imbriano LJ, Ilamathi E, Ali NM, Miyawaki N, & Maesaka JK. (2011) Normal fractional urate excretion identifies hyponatremic patients with reset osmostat (J. Nephrol In Press)

Jaenike JR, & Waterhouse C. (1961) The renal response to sustained administration of vasopressin and water in man. *J Clin Endocrinol Metab*,21,PP.231-242

Jensen KT, Carstens J, & Pedersen EB. (1998) Effect of BNP on renal hemodynamics, tubular function and vasoactive hormones in humans, *Am J Physiol*,274, pp. F63-F72.

Kahn T. (2003) Reset Osmostat and salt and water retention in the course of severe hyponatremia. *Medicine*,82,pp.170-176

Kasa M, Bierma TJ, Waterstraat F Jr, Corsaut M, & Singh SP. (1989) Routine blood chemistry screen: a diagnostic aid for Alzheimer's disease. *Neuroepidemiology*,8(5)pp.254-256

Leaf A, Bartter FC, Santos RF, & Wrong O. (1953) Evidence in man that urinary electrolyte loss induced by pitressin is a function of water retention. *J Clin Invest*,32,pp.868-878.

Leyssac PP, Holstein-Rathlou NH, Skøtt P, & Alfrey AC. (1990) A micropuncture study of proximal tubular transport of lithium during osmotic diuresis. *Am J Physiol*,258(4 Pt 2),pp.F1090-F1095.

Maack T, Marion DN, Camargo MJ, Kleinert HD, Laragh JH, & Vaughan ED Jr. (1984) Atlas SA: Effects of auriculin (atrial natriuretic factor) on blood pressure, renal function, and the renin-aldosterone system in dogs. *Am J Med*,77(6),pp.1069-1075.

Maesaka JK, & Fishbane S. (1998) Regulation of renal urate excretion: a critical review. *Am J Kidney Dis*,32,pp.917-933

Maesaka JK, Batuman V, Yudd M, Sale M, Sved AF, & Venkatesan J. (1990) Hyponatremia and hypouricemia: Differentiation from the syndrome of inappropriate secretion of antidiuretic hormone. *Clin Nephrol*,33,PP.174-178

Maesaka JK, Cusano AJ, Thies HL, Siegal FP, & Dreisbach A. (1990) Hypouricemia in acquired immunodeficiency syndrome. *Am. J. Kidney Dis*,15,pp.252-257

Maesaka JK, Gupta S, & Fishbane S. Cerebral salt wasting syndrome: does it exist? *Nephron* 82:100-109, 1999

Maesaka JK, Imbriano L, Ali N, & Ilamathi E. (2009) Mini Review. Is it cerebral or renal salt wasting? *Kidney Int*,76,pp.934-938

Maesaka JK, Miyawaki N, Palaia T, Fishbane S, & Durham J. (2007) Renal salt wasting without cerebral disease: value of determining urate in hyponatremia. *Kidney Int*,71,pp.822-826

Maesaka JK, Venkatesan J, Piccione JM, Decker R. Dreisbach AW, & Wetherington J. (1993) Plasma natriuretic factor(s) in patients with intracranial disease, renal salt wasting and hyperuricosuria. *Life Sci*,52,pp.1875-1882

Maesaka JK, Venkatesan J, Piccione JM, et al. (1992) Abnormal renal urate transport in patients with intracranial disease. *Am J Kidney Dis*,19,pp.10-15

Maesaka JK, Wolf-Klein G, Piccione JM, & Ma CM. (1993) Hyporuicemia, abnormal renal tubular urate transport, and plasma natriuretic factor(s) in patients with Alzheimer's disease. *J Am Geriatr Soc*, 41,pp.501-506

Maesaka JK. (1996) An expanded view of SIADH, hyponatremia, and hypouricemia. Editorial. *Clin Neph*,46,pp.79-83

Marik PE, Baram M, & Vahid B. (2008) Does central venous pressure predict fluid responsiveness? A systematic review of the literature and the tale of seven mares. *Chest*,134,pp.172-178

McCance RA. (1936) Experimental sodium chloride deficiency in man. *Proc Roy Soc, London*, ser. B 119,pp.245-268, 1936.

Milionis HJ, Kakafika Al, Tsouli SG, Athyros VG, Bairaktari ET, Seferiadis KI, & Elisaf MS.(2004) Effects of statin treatment on uric acid homeostasis in patient with primary hyperlipidemia. *Am. Heart J*, 148,pp. 635-640

Mulatero P, Rabbia F, Milan A, Paglieri C, Morello F, Chiandussi L, & Veglio F. (2002) Drug effects on aldosterone/plasma renin activity ratio in primary aldosteronism. *Hypertension*, 40,pp.897-902

Nelson PB, Seif SM, Maroon JC, & Robinson AG. (1981) Hyponatremia in intracranial disease: Perhaps not the syndrome of inappropriate secretion of antidiuretic hormone (SIADH). *J Neurosurg*,55,pp.938-941

Oh MS, & Carroll HS. (1999) Cerebral salt-wasting syndrome, we need better proof of its existence. *Nephron*, 82,pp.110-114

Oliver WJ, Cohen EL, & Neel JV. (1975) Blood pressure, sodium intake, and sodium related hormones in the Yanomamo Indians, a "No-Salt" culture. Circulation,52,pp.146-151.

Palmer BF. (2003) Hyponatremia in patients with central nervouos system disease: SIADH versus CSW. *Trends endocrinol metab*,14,pp.182-187

Passamonte PM. (1984) Hypouricemia, inappropriate secretion of antidiuretic hormone, and small cell carcinoma of the lung. *Arch Int Med*,144,pp.1569-1570

Peters JP, Welt LG, Sims EAH, Orloff J, & Needham J. (1950) A salt-wasting syndrome associated with cerebral disease. *Trans Assoc Am Physicians* 63,pp. 57-64

Ramsdell CM, & Kelley WN. (1973) The clinical significance of hypouricemia. *Ann Intern Med*,78,pp.239-242.

Renneboog B, Musch W, Vandemergel X, Mantu MU,& Cedaux G. (2006) Mild chronic hyponatremia is associated with falls, unsteadiness, and attention deficits. *Am J Med*,119,pp.711-718.

Richards AM, & Crozier IG. (1989) Physiological role of atrial natriuretic peptide. *Int J Cardiol*, 25,pp.141-144.

Robertson GL, & Ganguly A. (1986) Osmoregulation and baroregulation of plasma vasopressin in essential hypertension. *Cardiovasc Pharmacol*,8 Suppl 7,pp.S87-S91.

Roch-Ramel F, Guisan B.,& Schild L. (1996) Indirect coupling of urate and p-aminohippurate transport to sodium in human brush-border membrane vesciles. *Am J Physiol*,270,pp.F761-F68

Schneditz D. (2006) The arrow of bioimpedance. *Kidney Int*,69,pp.1492-1493

Schrier R. (2010) Does 'asymptomatic hyponatremia' exist? Nat Rev Nephrol,6,pp.1

Schrier RW, Gross P, Gheorghiade M, Berl T, Verbalis JG, Czerwiec FS, & Orlandi C; SALT Investigators. (2006)Tolvaptan, a selective oral vasopressin V2-receptor antagonist, for hyponatremia. *N Engl J Med*,355, pp. 2099-112

Schwartz WB, Bennett W, & Curelop S. (1957) A syndrome of renal sodium loss and hyponatremia probably resulting from inappropriate secretion of antidiuretic hormone. *Am J Med*,23,pp.529-542

Shannon JA. (1936) Glomerular filtration and urea excretion in relation to urine flow in the dog. *Am J Physiol*,117,pp.206-225.

Sherlock M, O'Sullivan E, Agha A, Behan LA, Rawluk D, Brennan P, Tormey W, & Thompson CJ. (2006) The incidence and pathophysiology of hyponatremia in subarachnoid hemorrhage. *Clin Endocrinol*,64,pp.250-254

Sherlock M, O'Sullivan E, Agba A,k Behan LA, Owens D, Finucane F, Rawluck D, Tormey W, & Thompson CJ. (2009) Incidence and pathophysiology of severe hyponatremia in neurosurgical patients. *Postgrad Med*,85,pp.171-175

Sing S, Bohn D, Cariotti AP, Cusimano M, Rutka JT, & Halperin ML. (2002) Cerebral salt wasting: Truths, fallacies, theories, and challenges. *Crit Care Med*,30,pp.2575-2579

Sivakumar V, Rajshekhar V, & Chandy MJ. (1994) Management of neurosurgical patient with hyponatremia and natriuresis. *Neurosurgery*,43,pp.269-274

Sonnenblick M, & Rosin A. (1988) Increased uric acid clearance in the syndrome of inappropriate secretion of antidiuretic hormone. *Isr J Med Sci*,24,pp.20-23

Sonnenblick M, & Rosin AJ. (1986) Significance of the measurement of uric acid fractional clearance in diuretic induced hyponatremia. *Postgrad Med* J,62(728),pp.449-452

Sorensen JB, Osterlind K, Kristiansen PEG, Hammer M, & Hansen M. (1988) Hypouricemia and urate excretion in small cell lung carcinoma patients with syndrome of inappropriate antidiuresis. *Acta Oncol*,27,pp.351-355.

Steele A, Gowrishankar M, Abrahamson S, Mazer CD, Feldman RD, & Halperin ML. (1997) Postoperative hyponatremia despite near-isotonic saline infusion: a phenomenon of desalination. *Ann Intern Med*,126,pp.20-25

Steele T. (1969) Evidence for altered renal urate reabsorption during changes in volume of the extracellular fluid. *J Lab Clin Med*,74,pp.288-299

Steele TH. Oppenheimer S: Factors affecting urate excretion following diuretic administration in man. *Am J Med* 1969; 47: 564-574

Sterns RH, & Silver SM. (2008) Cerebral salt wasting versus SIADH: what difference? *J Am Soc Nephrol*,18(2),pp.194-196

Sterns RH, Nigwekar SU, & Hix JK. (2009) The treatment of hyponatremia. *Sem Nephrol*,29(3),pp.282-299.

Strauss MB, Lamdin E, Smith P, & Bleifer DJ. (1958) Surfeit and deficit of sodium. *Arch Int Med*,102,pp.527-536.

Traynor TR, Smart A, Briggs JP, & Schnermann J. (1999) Inhibition of macula densa-stimulated renin secretion by pharmacological blockade of cyclooxygenase-2. *Am J Physiol*,277(5 Pt 2),pp.F706-F710.

Valtin H: (1997) Renal dysfunction: Disorders of Na+ balance. Edema first edition: Mechanism involved in the fluid and solute imbalance. Little Brown and company (Inc), Boston,pp.58-59.

Verbalis JG, Adler S, Schrier RW, Berl T, Zhao Q, & Czerwiec FS: SALT Investigators. (2011) Efficacy and safety of oral tolvaptan therapy in patients with the syndrome of inappropriate antidiuretic hormone secretion. Eur J Endocrinol 164,pp. 725-732

Verbalis JG, Goldsmith SR, Greenberg A, Schrier RW, & Sterns RH. (2007) Hyponastremia treatment guidelines 2007: Expert Panel Recommendations. *Am J Med,*120,pp.S1-S21

Vogel JH. (1963) Aldosterone in the cerebral salt wasting. *Circulation,*127,pp.44-50.

Wall BM, Crofton JT, & Share L. (1992) Chronic hyponatremia due to resetting of the osmostat in a patient with gastric carcinoma. *Am J Med* 1992,93,pp.223-228

Wall BM. (1993) Water loading test in the reset osmostat variant of SIADH. *Am J Med.*94,pp.343.

Weinberger A, Santo M, Solomon F, Shalit M, Pinkhas J, & Sperling O. (1982) Abnormality in renal urate handling in the syndrome of inappropriate secretion of antidiuretic hormone. *Isr J Med,*18,pp.711-713.

Welt LG, Seldin DW, Nelson WP, German WJ, & Peters JP. (1952) Role of the central nervous system in metabolism of electrolytes and water. *Arch Int Med,*90,pp.355-378)

Wijdicks EF, Ropper AH, Hunnicutt EJ, Richardson GS, & Nathanson JA. (1991) Atrial natriuretic factor and salt wasting after aneurysmal subarachnoid hemorrhage. *Stroke,*22(12),pp.1519-1524.

Wijdicks EF, Schievink WI,& Burnett JC Jr. (1997) Natriuretic peptide system and endothelin in aneurysmal subarachnoid hemorrhage. *J Neurosurg,* 87(2),pp.275-80 (ANP)

Wijdicks EF, Vermeulen M, Haaf JA, Hijdra A, Bakker WH, van Gijn J. (1985) Volume depletion and natriuresis in patients with a ruptured intracranial aneurysm. *Ann Neurol,*18,pp.211-216

Wijdicks EF, Vermeulen M, Hijdra A, & van Gijn J. (1985) Hyponatremia and cerebral infarction in patients with ruptured intracranial aneurysm: Is fluid restriction harmful. *Ann Neurol,*17,PP.137-140

Yamamoto T, Moriwaki Y, Takahashi S, Tsutsumi Z, & Hada T. (2000) Effect of losartan potassium, an angiotensin II receptor antagonist, on renal excretion of oxypurinol and purine bases. *J Rheumatol,* 27,pp. 2232-2236

Youmans S, & Maesaka JK.(2011) Urine of patients with cerebral/renal salt-wasting syndrome contains a substance that inhibits reabsorptive sodium flux in LLC-PK1 cellsAbst. *Annual Mtg Am Soc Nephrol,* Philadelphia, PA, USA

Zerbe R, Stropes L, & Robertson G. (1980) Vasopressin function in the syndrome of inappropriate antidiuresis. *Annu Rev Med,* 31,pp.315-327

4

Epidemiology, Causes and Outcome of Obstetric Acute Kidney Injury

Namrata Khanal[1*], Ejaz Ahmed[2] and Fazal Akhtar[2]
[1]Middlemore Hospital, Auckland,
[2]Department of Renal Medicine,
Sindh Institute of Urology and Transplantation, Karachi,
[1]New Zealand
[2]Pakistan

1. Introduction

Acute kidney injury (AKI) is a clinical syndrome denoted by an abrupt decline in glomerular filtration rate (GFR) sufficient to decrease the elimination of nitrogenous waste products (urea and creatinine) and other uremic toxins (Jefferson et al, 2010). AKI is a not very common yet serious complication occurring in pregnancy. The incidence and the mortality rates associated with obstetric acute kidney injury (also known as pregnancy related acute renal failure; PRARF) have decreased over the last few decades especially in developed countries (Prakash et al, 2007; Stratta et al, 1996). There are several factors which lead to this improvement and will be discussed later in the chapter. Since the term AKI is now widely used in place of acute renal failure (Ricci et al, 2011); for the ease of description we have used obstetric AKI in place of PRARF in this chapter.

Obstetric AKI can occur at any stage of pregnancy; ante-partum or post-partum and may be AKI occurring as a coincidence during pregnancy or AKI due to causes specific to pregnancy.

Although obstetric AKI is vanishing from developed world (Stratta et al, 1996), it is still a frequent cause of maternal morbidity and mortality in the developing nations. Poverty, lack of awareness and difficulties (e.g. lack of transport) accessing obstetric care all are responsible for this additional burden (World Health Organization [WHO], 2009). This also increases the disparity in reported number of cases and its actual occurrence contributing to scarcity of literature even in recent time.

1.1 Definition and epidemiology of Acute Kidney Injury (AKI) and obstetric AKI

Insight into the occurrence and consequences of kidney disease has rapidly progressed. More than 30 different definitions have been used for defining AKI in the literature, creating much confusion and making comparisons difficult (Bellomo et al, 2001). Recently, consensus

---

* Corresponding Author

definitions and classification systems have been proposed for AKI. RIFLE criteria stratify AKI into five stages (Table 1). This will eventually allow consistency across studies such that results can be compared (Ricci et al, 2011).

System	Serum creatinine criteria	Urine output criteria
RIFLE class		
Risk	Serum creatinine increase to 1.5-fold OR GFR decrease >25% from baseline	<0.5 ml/kg/h for 6 h
Injury	Serum creatinine increase to 2.0-fold OR GFR decrease >50% from baseline	<0.5 ml/kg/h for 12 h
Failure	Serum creatinine increase to 3.0-fold OR GFR decrease >75% from baseline OR serum creatinine ≥354 µmol/l (≥4 mg/dl) with an acute increase of at least 44 µmol/l (0.5 mg/dl)	Anuria for 12 h
AKIN Stage		
1	Serum creatinine increase ≥26.5 µmol/l (≥0.3 mg/dl) OR increase to 1.5–2.0-fold from baseline	<0.5 ml/kg/h for 6 h
2	Serum creatinine increase >2.0–3.0-fold from baseline	<0.5 ml/kg/h for 12 h
3	Serum creatinine increase >3.0-fold from baseline OR serum creatinine ≥354 µmol/l (≥4.0 mg/dl) with an acute increase of at least 44 µmol/l (0.5 mg/dl) OR need for RRT	<0.3 ml/kg/h for 24 h OR anuria for 12 h OR need for RRT

Small but important differences are observed between the two systems. A time constraint of 48 h for diagnosis (using either serum creatinine levels or urine output) is required in AKIN criteria. GFR decreases are used for diagnosis only in RIFLE criteria. In both systems, only one criterion (creatinine or urine output) has to be met to qualify for a given class or stage of AKI. Classes L and E of the RIFLE criteria are not reported. Owing to the wide variation in indications for and timing of initiation of RRT, individuals who receive RRT are considered to have AKIN Stage 3 AKI irrespective of their serum creatinine level and urine output.6,15 Abbreviations: AKI, acute kidney injury; AKIN, AKI Network; GFR, glomerular filtration rate; RIFLE, Risk, Injury Failure, Loss, End-stage renal disease; RRT, renal replacement therapy.

Table 1. Classification and staging systems for AKI.

AKI is estimated to occur in as many as 4%-20% of hospital admissions (Waikar et al, 2008) and in approximately 5-6% of critically ill patients with the period prevalence ranging from 1-25% (Uchino et al, 2005). Similarly, the period prevalence for acute renal replacement therapy in ICU is around 4-5% (Uchino et al, 2005). Septic shock in itself attributes to 50-60% of the cases. Hospital mortality in critically ill patients with AKI is equally higher at approximately 60% and has been reported to range from 28-90% (Uchino et al, 2005; Bellomo et al, 2004).

Incidence of pregnancy related AKI used to be 24-40% of all AKI in 60's which decreased to 2-3% in 80's (Fig 1) (Stratta, 1996). Interestingly enough, its incidence was already decreasing in 1963 as compared to 1959 when AKI occurred in 1 in 5000 pregnancies and 1 in 1400 pregnancies respectively in developed countries (Smith et al, 1965; Knapp & Hellman, 1959).

The incidence of obstetric AKI has further declined over last 4 decades (Prakash et al, 2010). This improvement is due to improved availability of safe and legal abortion, more widespread and aggressive antibiotic use decreasing the incidence of post-abortal sepsis, and improved prenatal care. In the past, obstetric AKI used to be mostly due to post-abortal sepsis (Gul et al, 2004). Four decade long retrospective review of pregnancy related AKI cases was published from a centre in Italy. They reported virtual non-existence of post abortal sepsis, while AKI from obstetric complications like amniotic fluid embolism, extensive haemorrhage and prolonged intrauterine death etc. had decreased. AKI associated with preeclampsia and eclampsia remained stable until 1987 however its incidence decreased dramatically thereafter contributing towards the improved maternal mortality rate. The decreased occurrence was more evident in developed nations (Stratta et al, 1996). In 1995, the maternal mortality ratio in Africa was estimated to be over 1000 per 100 000 pregnancies and in Europe 28 per 100 000 pregnancies (Hill et al., 2001). In a recent review on AKI amongst all hospital admissions, pregnancy related AKI has not been listed as one of the causes of AKI. Authors have included critically ill patients with AKI in this review and have reviewed around 170 published literatures (Waikar et al, 2008). It may not be an over statement to say that these cases are declining in incidence furthermore.

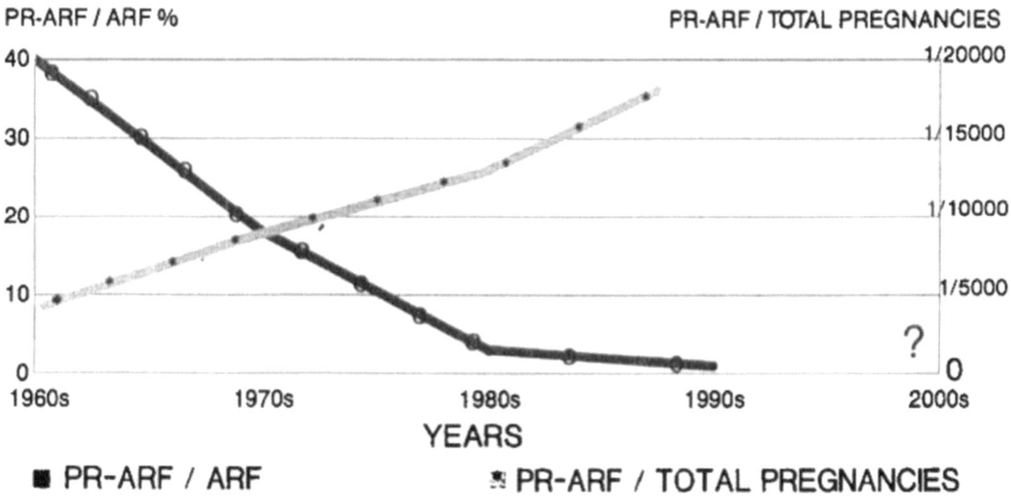

Fig. 1. Incidence of pregnancy related AKI.

However in recent reports published from developing countries; the frequency of obstetric AKI have been reported to be varying between 4-15% (Sivakumar et al, 2011). In a single centre study from India the incidence of AKI was reported as 1 in 56 births (Prakash et al, 2010) in contrast to 1 in 20000 births as reported from Italy (Stratta et al, Ren Fail 1996). Similar studies from individual centre from various developing countries have been published over the last decade emphasizing the fact that obstetric AKI is still prevalent in the developing or poor income nations (Table 2). However due to the absence of meta-analysis on obstetric AKI especially from these countries it is difficult to precisely estimate its actual incidence.

Author	Year published	Study popn	Obs-AKI (%)	Septic abortion	APH/ PPH	Pre Eclampsia/ HELLP	DIC	Puerperal sepsis	Misc.
Chugh et al	1976	325	22.1	31	12	8	9	9	12
Prakash et al	1995	426	13.9	45	2	4	-	5	3
*Prakash et al	2006	190	-	130	11	33	-	16	-
Kilari et al	2006	41	4.24	4	7	10	-	12	8
Goplani et al	2008	70	9.06	14	27	20	23	43	17
Saleem Najar et al	2008	40	7.02	20	8	6	4	-	6
Hassan et al	2009	130	33	-	24	5	4	12	-
*Khalil et al	2009	60	-	3	22	10	11	1	4
*Khanal et al	2010	50	-	3	36	14	-	16	18
Prakash et al	2010	106	20.75	Only included patients with preeclampsia					
**Prakash et al	2010	4758	1.78	NA	16	30	14	21	18
Agida et al	2010	46	13	Only included patients with preeclampsia					
*Erdemoglu et al	2010	75	-	11	9	57	-	-	-
Sivakumar et al	2011	59	4.36	28	11	18	-	-	11

* Study population included all pregnant women with AKI, causes listed existed together or individually **only included patients in third trimester; NA: not applicable; this series had sepsis as cause of AKI in 16 (18.8%) patients

Table 2. Incidence and causes of Obstetric AKI in developing countries.

1.2 Causes of AKI (Table 3)

First of all, any cause which can give rise to AKI in non-pregnant women of reproductive age group (pre-renal, renal, and post renal or obstructive) may contribute to AKI in pregnancy. They can be coincidental simultaneous occurrences in pregnant women. As in any evaluation of AKI, causes not related to pregnancy must thus be considered and excluded. Pregnancy unrelated causes of AKI represent only about 5% of all obstetric AKI (Krane, 1988).

A second group of patients are those with underlying chronic renal disease that worsens during pregnancy, suggesting the development of acute renal failure superimposed on their chronic diseases. Glomerular diseases might be diagnosed for the first time in pregnancy and AKI may occur as a result of rapidly progressive glomerulonephritis. Examples of disorders that may show a decline in the GFR include chronic glomerular diseases, lupus nephritis, diabetic nephropathy, and the chronic interstitial nephritides. Discussion on renal function during pregnancy in women with underlying renal disease is beyond the scope of this chapter.

Finally, there are causes of renal failure specific to pregnancy, which are relatively more commonly encountered in gravid women. AKI seems to have bimodal distribution during pregnancy in first trimester and third trimester respectively.

Acute renal Failure in During early pregnancy
•Acute or massive blood loss
-Abortion
-Ectopic
-Hyaditiform mole
•Severe dehydration
-Ac. Pyelonephritis
-Hyperemesis gravidarum
• ATN resulting from a septic abortion
ARF Late in Pregnancy/Postpartum
•Thrombotic microangiopathy
-TTP-HUS
-Severe preeclampsia usually with HELLP syndrome
•Renal Cortical Necrosis resulting from
-Placenta previa
-Prolonged intrauterine foetal death
-Amniotic fluid embolism
•Intrinsic renal disease/autoimmune diseases
•Acute pyelonephritis
-ATN from septicaemia or hypotension
-ARF from micro abscesses
•Acute fatty liver of pregnancy
Obstructive Causes
-Mild-moderate hydronephrosis is normal
-Occasionally, degree of obstruction sufficient to cause ARF
-Nephrolithiasis if solitary functioning kidney

Table 3. Causes of Acute kidney Injury in Pregnancy.

Prerenal azotemia is the most common cause of both community and hospital-acquired AKI. It is an appropriate physiological response to renal hypo perfusion (Blantz, 1998). Similarly, the most common cause of AKI specifically in first trimester of pregnancy is prerenal azotemia owing to hyperemesis gravidarum or vomiting from acute pyelonephritis. In late pregnancy volume contraction may be secondary to blood loss (Pertuiset & Grunfled, 1994). Antepartum and postpartum haemorrhage have been reported as major causes of AKI in pregnancy (Smith et al, 1965; Kennedy et al, 1973; Ali et al, 2004). Pregnant women who sustained AKI receive blood transfusion frequently; this further emphasizes the frequency of significant haemorrhage in these patients (Ali et al, 2004; Khanal et al, 2010). Uterine bleeding secondary to abortion or septic abortions are still chief causes of obstetric AKI in developing countries.

Pregnancy-specific conditions such as preeclampsia, HELLP syndrome, acute fatty liver of pregnancy (AFLP), haemolytic uremic syndrome/ thrombotic thrombocytopenic purpura independently or in combination cause uterine bleeding ante-partum or post-partum haemorrhage. These conditions are frequently associated with complications like abruptio-placentae, hepatic infarction, hepatic rupture, intra-abdominal bleeding, and puerperal sepsis all of which can be further complicated by AKI. This occurs frequently in third trimester (Krane, 1988; Maynard et al, 2007; Prakash, 2010). Preeclampsia is a multi-system disorder unique to human pregnancy characterised by hypertension and involvement of one or more other organ systems and/or the foetus. American College of Obstetrics and Gynaecology, requires blood pressures >140/90 mm Hg on two occasions combined with urinary protein excretion >300 mg/d for the diagnosis of preeclampsia. Preeclampsia occurs in 3-5% of pregnancies and is associated with increased maternal and fetal mortality especially in developing countries. It is a leading cause of premature deliveries in developed countries thus increases the neonatal morbidity (Society of Obstetric Medicine of Australia and New Zealand [SOMANZ], 2009).

Abruptio placentae and puerperal sepsis; may also occur independent of these conditions and can be complicated by AKI. Obstetric complications such as septic abortion and placental abruption are associated with severe acute tubular necrosis (ATN) and bilateral cortical necrosis. Acute cortical necrosis, usually involves bilateral renal cortex, may occur as a consequence of irreversible or severe ATN. It has been found to be associated with poor renal outcome in longer term. Bilateral cortical necrosis is most often a complication of abruptio-placentae (36 per cent in the series of Chugh); while in other studies it was associated with disseminated intravascular coagulation. It presents as acute renal failure in other conditions too but, unlike acute tubular necrosis, total and persistent anuria is almost constant (Kleinknecht et al, 1973; Chugh, 1976). The diagnosis can be established either by renal biopsy or, better, by selective renal angiography. Other imaging studies (plain radiograph, ultrasound scan, CT-scan of abdomen and nuclear renal scan) may also be helpful. Renal cortical necrosis which occurs as a consequence of AKI in pregnancy continues sporadically (Naqvi et al, 1996; Prakash et al, 2007). With overall decrease in the incidence of AKI in pregnancy and improved overall management; incidence of cortical necrosis is decreasing even in the developing countries. Whenever present it is associated with irreversible renal failure (Khanal, 2010). Sepsis is still a major cause including septic abortions and puerperal sepsis in several studies published from India over last decades (Sivakumar, 2011).

Less common and miscellaneous causes of obstetric AKI include:

Obstructive uropathy; obstruction may occur in gravidas due to polyhydramnios, incarcerated gravid uterus, or can occur even in women with otherwise uncomplicated gestation due to retroverted uterus. Rarely, acute urinary tract obstruction in pregnancy is induced by a kidney stone, and it seldom causes renal failure (Strothers & Lee, 1992; Scarpa et al, 1996).

Amniotic fluid embolism which occurs primarily in multi-para after prolonged labour can cause AKI. Those with underlying renal parenchymal disease even without advanced chronic kidney disease are more prone to develop acute tubular necrosis (ATN) especially due to super imposed pre-eclampsia (Pertuiset & Grunfeld, 1994). Thrombotic thrombocytopenic purpura-haemolytic uremic syndrome (TTP-HUS) can easily be confused with severe preeclampsia, usually with the HELLP syndrome (haemolysis with a microangiopathic blood smear, elevated liver enzymes, and a low platelet count) (McCrae et al, 1992) both can cause AKI.

There are anecdotal reports on sporadic cases of acute glomerulonephritis (GN) including post infectious GN, good-pasture's syndrome, lymphoma, drug nephrotoxicity, incompatible blood transfusions and endocarditis causing AKI during pregnancy (Pertuiset & Grunfeld, 1994). Acute interstitial nephritis (from antibiotics or non-steroidal anti-inflammatory drugs etc.) may coincidentally occur during pregnancy and result in AKI.

1.3 Changes in renal anatomy and physiology in normal pregnancy:

To understand the pathophysiology and proper management of renal problems in pregnancy it is important that we are familiar with the anatomical and physiological changes that occur during normal pregnancy.

1.3.1 Renal tract anatomy

The kidneys enlarge during normal pregnancy, increasing by 1 to 2 cm in length and in volume by up to 70% towards term, due to tissue hypertrophy and expansion of both interstitial and vascular compartments. More important from a clinical perspective is the increase in size of the renal pelvices and ureters. By third trimester about 80% of the pregnant women have hydronephrosis which is easily evident by ultrasound, more on the right than on the left (Baylis & Davison , 2010; Brown et al, 2010). A number of factors are thought to be important in this change. Progesterone, a smooth muscle relaxant, reduces ureteric tone and peristalsis. The asymmetric dilation of the pelvicalyceal system suggests extrinsic compression by the enlarging uterus at the pelvic brim, hypertrophy of surrounding connective tissue (Waldeyer's sheath) and kinking due to ligaments or compression by iliac blood vessels (Brown et al, 2010). The clinical consequence of these changes can be urinary stasis; increasing the risk of bacterial growth and asymptomatic bacteriuria of pregnancy. If the changes are in extreme and precipitate the over distention syndrome, with massive dilation they may present with symptoms like recurrent severe flank pain, increasing serum creatinine, hypertension, or even reversible acute kidney injury (Khanna & Nguyen, 2001). In case of presentation with over distension symptoms that suggest renal colic but no stone detectable by ultrasound or by radiographic imaging; it is imperative to exclude urinary tract infection and to avoid the temptation to drain the system using nephrostomy tubes. Furthermore it is important to remember that acute renal failure as a consequence of ureteric obstruction in pregnancy is uncommon; and that ureteric dilation is part of normal pregnancy and it is not usually possible to distinguish between this and pathologic dilation (Brown et al, 2010).

1.3.2 Renal physiology

1.3.2.1 Systemic haemodynamics

Detailed discussion of systemic haemodynamics of normal pregnancy is beyond the scope of this chapter. Briefly, changes start as early as the first trimester with reduced systemic vascular resistance, increase in cardiac output by 40-50% and resting tachycardia by 24th week (Davison & Dunlop, 1980). There is progressive expansion of the plasma and extracellular fluid volume, reaching a maximum of 1.25 litres at times. The volume of the total extracellular fluid space is determined principally by sodium and hence water accumulation. The combination of increased cardiac output and peripheral vasodilatation means that organ blood flow increases in pregnancy, with the most dramatic changes occurring in the kidney and skin circulation throughout gestation and in the uterus in the second part of the pregnancy. These changes result in a small reduction in arterial blood pressure, typically reaching a nadir in the mid-trimester of about 10 mmHg systolic, rising towards pre-pregnancy levels at term (Brown & Gallery, 1994). Table 4 illustrates changes in some common indices during pregnancy.

	Non-Pregnant	Pregnant
Hematocrit (%)	41	33
Plasma creatinine (μmol/L)	<120	<90
mg/dl	<1.3	<1
Plasma urea (mmol/L)	11.2-31	9-12
mg/dl	4-11	3.2-4.4
Plasma albumin (g/L)	35-45	25-35
(g/dl)	3.5-4.5	2.5-3.5
Plasma uric acid mg/dl (μmol/L)	4 (240)	3.2 (190) early
		4.3 (260) late
Plasma bicarbonate (mmol/l, meq/l)	22-28	18-20
Urinary protein excretion (mg/d)	<150	<300

Table 4. Changes in some common indices during pregnancy (Modified from Source: Baylis & Davison, 2010; Brown et al 2010).

1.3.2.2 Renal haemodynamics

There is approximately 25% increase in glomerular filtration rate (GFR) by 4 weeks. This reaches a nadir of ~50% by mid pregnancy and is maintained until the last few weeks of pregnancy after which it starts to decrease however still remaining above the non-pregnant level. This leads to fall in serum creatinine (see Table 4). More pronounced is the increased renal plasma flow and decline in filtration fraction; both return to non pregnant level towards the term (Baylis & Davison, 2010).

In pre-eclampsia both renal plasma flow (RPF) and GFR decreases. There is salt retention and contraction of plasma volume as compared to normal pregnancy (Brown & Gallery, 1994). Although the absolute values of RPF and GFR may remain above non-pregnant level, this is probably the most likely mechanism of hypofiltration in this condition. The endothelium is involved inclusive of glomerulus, causing vascular endothelial cell dysfunction (glomerular endotheliosis) and results in swollen bloodless glomeruli and the loss of glomerular barrier size and charge selectivities (Baylis & Davison, 2010). This pattern is also seen in normal pregnancy and not pathognomonic of pre-eclampsia (Strevens, 2003).

1.3.3 Pathophysiology of AKI in preeclampsia/ eclampsia and other microangiopathies

In severe pre-eclampsia/ eclampsia, renal failure is most probably due to acute tubular necrosis (Sibai et al, 1993). ATN in these women is frequently due to haemorrhage; for reasons explained in previous sections. AKI may also complicate postpartum eclampsia. HELLP syndrome (haemolysis, elevated liver enzymes and low platelet count) is a variant of severe pre-eclampsia, which usually resolves following delivery (Weinstein, 1985) and occurs in around 20% of the severe pre-eclampsia cases (Sibai et al, 1993). AKI may also occur as a direct consequence of disseminated intravascular coagulation (one of the dreaded complications in upto 20% of women with HELLP syndrome), and sepsis (Sibai et al, 1993).

Similarly, other microangiopathies like acute fatty liver of pregnancy which occurs commonly in the third trimester and haemolytic uremic syndrome/ thrombotic thrombocytopenic purpura occurring ante- or post-partum share several pathophysiologic mechanisms which is difficult to differentiate and eventually may contribute to the development of AKI (Ganesan, 2011). Acute fatty liver of pregnancy is an obstetric emergency, which if untreated may progress to fulminant hepatic failure and proves life threatening to both mother and foetus. Variable degree of AKI has been reported in upto 90% of women with acute fatty liver of pregnancy, which is usually reversible with the recovery of liver failure (Hou, 2001). HUS/TTP occurs typically in the early postpartum period but delays of several months postpartum have also been reported. Renal failure was previously thought to be irreversible but complete and partial recovery does occur in about 30% of these cases (Beaufils, 2001).

1.3.4 Pyelonephritis, septic abortion and puerperal sepsis

Pathogenesis of sepsis-induced renal dysfunction is still poorly understood. Though it has been demonstrated that septic AKI can occur in the setting of marked Hyperaemia and vasodilatation; and renal ischemia is not necessary for the loss of GFR (Bellomo et al, 2008); various inflammatory factors have also been shown to be generated following ischemia which contributes to development of AKI and ATN (Kribben, 1999). Experimental studies continue to report newer concepts for pathogenesis of septic AKI (Bellomo, 2011). Similar studies in man are required to confirm these experimental findings.

Pregnant women are at greater risk of urinary tract infection due to the altered anatomy and urinary stasis as discussed in previous sections. Untreated timely and correctly this can lead to urosepsis. Acute pyelonephritis may occur as part of urinary tract infection and may be severe enough to cause AKI as a result of sepsis or prerenal azotemia from vomiting. Improved availability and better management of abortion has led to decrease in the incidence of post-abortal sepsis especially in the developed countries (Gul et al, 2004). Sepsis is still a major cause including septic abortions and puerperal sepsis in developing countries (Sivakumar, 2011; Khanal, 2010).

1.4 Prevention and model of care

A total of 99% of all maternal deaths occur in developing countries, where 85% of the population lives. More than half of these deaths occur in sub-Saharan Africa and one third in South Asia. Globally, around 80 per cent of maternal deaths are due to obstetric complications; mainly haemorrhage, sepsis, unsafe abortion, pre-eclampsia and eclampsia, and prolonged or obstructed labour (United Nations Children's Fund [UNICEF], 2003; United Nations Development Programme [UNDP], 2006). An estimated 21.6 million unsafe abortions took place worldwide in 2008, almost all in developing countries. Numbers of unsafe abortions have increased from 19.7 million in 2003 (Department of Reproductive

Health and Research, WHO, 2011). Complications of unsafe abortions account for 13 per cent of maternal deaths worldwide, and 19 per cent of maternal deaths in South America (Ahman et al 2002; WHO, 2004). Preeclampsia is associated with poor maternal outcome including maternal death even in developed countries (SOMANZ, 2009; Isler , 1999).

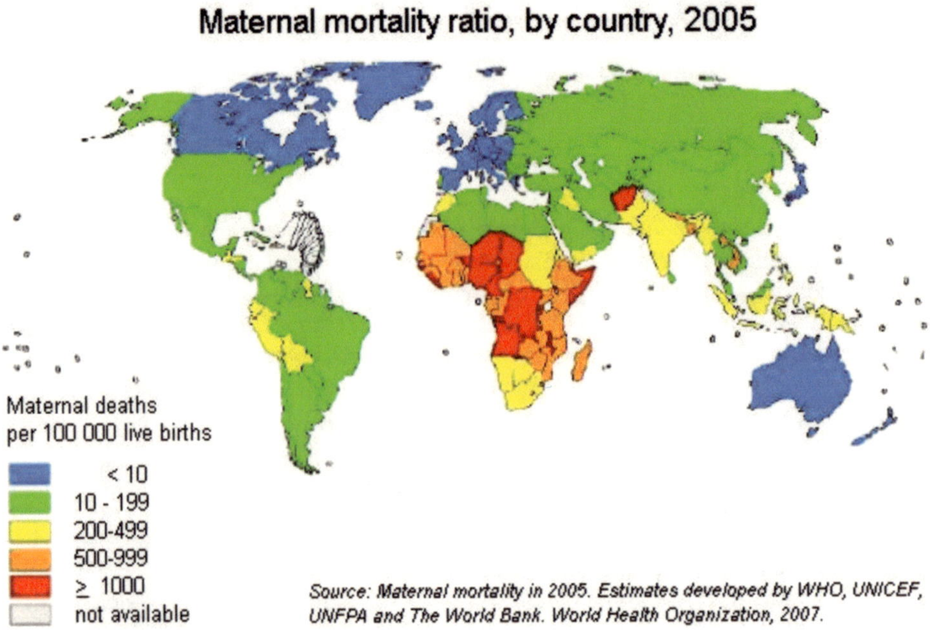

Fig. 2. Maternal mortality ratio by country.

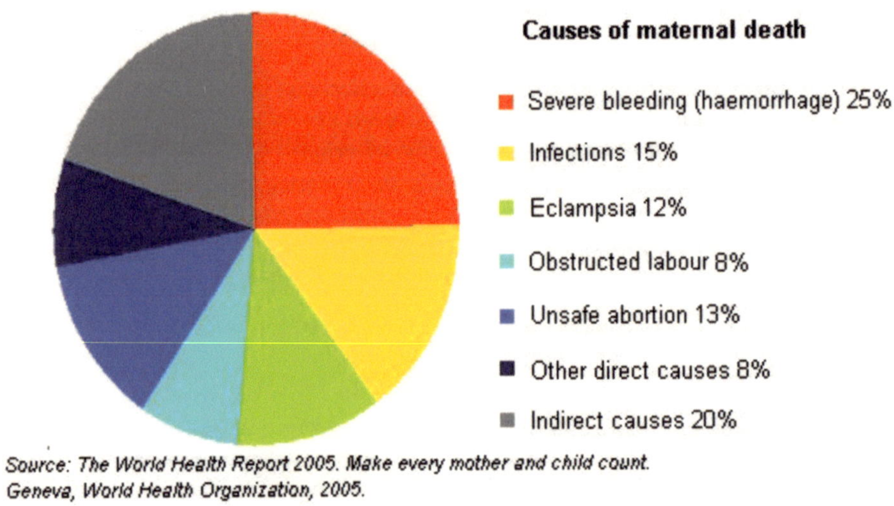

Fig. 3. Causes of maternal death.

One of the many complications contributing to this burden is AKI occurring as a consequence of these complications. It is very difficult to postulate any specific measure to prevent the occurrence of acute kidney injury. Adequate timely management of the underlying condition which may be complicated by AKI is the only way to prevent it from happening. The physiologic changes in renal system that occur with pregnancy increasing the risk of infection are in itself non-modifiable, so is preeclampsia. Acute on chronic deterioration of renal function can probably be prevented by selecting women who are at lowest risk of progression of their existing kidney disease and perhaps counselling others for contraception is the only solution. Hence development of model of care is of utmost importance to reduce the maternal/ foetal mortality and morbidity; as has been long recognized by WHO (WHO, 2011); which is probably made worse by poor renal outcome in pregnant mothers. Widespread availability of improved prenatal care through midwives and timely recognition/ referral of high risk cases have decreased the incidence of pregnancy related AKI in developed world. An estimated 74 per cent of maternal deaths could be averted if all women had access to the interventions for preventing or treating pregnancy and birth complications, in particular emergency obstetric care (Barbinard & Roberts, 2006). There is need to improve the provision of quality services in developing countries. Factors such as poverty, gender inequalities, illiteracy, poor health systems, political instability, cultural barriers, and lack of infrastructure (e.g. lack of transport) in certain areas making it difficult to access the facility all contribute to increased burden (WHO, 2011).

Measures to decrease maternal mortality also aim to reduce the consequences women face as a result of these complications. AKI is one of them. Below are our recommendations in keeping with the guidelines proposed by WHO and UNFPA (United Nations family planning association) in Millennium Summit as Millennium development goal 5 (MDG5) which will probably help to decrease maternal mortality in developing countries:

Firstly, it is very important for the pregnant women to understand the benefits of seeking safe abortion, utilizing antenatal follow up and when possible avoid unplanned pregnancies. It is likely that the morbidity and mortality risk would be reduced with adequate antenatal and delivery care (Robinson & Wharrad, 2001; de Bernis et al., 2000). **Secondly**, increasing the number of health personnel in form of midwives and trained birth attendants and making them available for these populations, frequent free health camps at remote areas to identify the population at risk e.g. identifying women with underlying kidney disease, and education on family planning and easy access to contraceptive measures, increasing its availability and legalizing the abortions are beneficial. **Finally**, timely intervention when needed through experts when needed for e.g. timely administration of antibiotics for infection, adequate management of hypovolaemia, performing caesarean section when indicated, and vigilant post partum care of these women all are important steps to prevent complication and thus reduce maternal mortality. Increased use of contraception has an obvious and direct effect on the maternal death rate per 1000 women of reproductive age and on the lifetime risk of maternal death, by reducing the number of pregnancies (Royston & Armstrong, 1989). Unsafe abortions are entirely preventable, and yet continue to occur in almost all developing countries and in Eastern Europe. The evidence suggests that this can be greatly reduced when (Department of Reproductive Health and Research, WHO, 2011):

- Pregnancies can be planned through effective contraception;
- Counselling and services meet the unmet need for family planning, and appropriate method mix of contraception is offered to all women, including both married and unmarried women; and

- Safe abortion services are available and accessible.

In the meantime ill-effects of unsafe abortion should be prevented by:

- making safe abortions services available and accessible where abortion is not against the law;
- ensuring that permitted reasons for abortion are supported by the national legislative process and health systems;
- granting access to services for the management of complications arising from unsafe abortion; and
- Providing post abortion counselling and offering contraceptive services, this will also help to avoid repeat abortion.

Similarly, preeclampsia occurs in 3-5% of pregnancies and is associated with increased maternal and foetal mortality especially in developing countries. If women with these problems are identified in antenatal period, safe delivery can be planned before hand (WHO, Dept. of Reproductive Health and Research, Dept. of Maternal, Newborn, Child and Adolescent Health, Dept. of Nutrition for Health and Development, 2011). Some reports have been published where the authors have questioned the importance of presence of skilled birth attendance at delivery and suggested that perhaps partnership between midwives and doctors and timely referral is more important to achieve this target (Cross et al, 2010) of reducing maternal mortality by 2/3 in these regions. Despite efforts from national, international and global health organizations MMR declined by only 5% from 1990-2005. To achieve this target of decline in MMR by 2/3 by 2015 will require tremendous work in this area. Any improvement in the maternal mortality rate will eventually lead to decrease consequences like AKI from various complications during pregnancy in developing countries.

1.5 Management outline

1.5.1 Fluid and electrolyte balance (Maynard et al, 2010)

Timely recognition of the events and adequate replenishment of the fluid volume is essential to prevent more dreaded complication of acute tubular necrosis (ATN). Eventually when AKI ensues management depends on the underlying cause of renal dysfunction. To avoid/ correct hypovolaemia and ascertain fluid balance is important at every stage. Where bleeding is the cause of hypovolaemia, measures to stop bleeding should precede all other procedures, this may necessitate termination of pregnancy, preterm delivery of the foetus and blood transfusion. Efforts should be made not to incite further insult by avoiding or minimising the use of nephrotoxic agents including radio-contrast dyes and various drugs as much as possible. If they have to be used; adjustment of the dose will be required. Equal attention has to be paid to ensure adequate electrolyte balance. Of all potassium requires regular monitoring. Hyperkalaemia demands urgent medical management and if persistent may be an indication for renal replacement therapy.

1.5.2 Appropriate management of sepsis

When infection coexists; use of appropriate antibiotics empirically is justified. Ensuring the safety of antibiotics during pregnancy is of utmost importance. Initial choice of antibiotics may vary according to the hospital protocol and prevalence of antibiotic resistance for the suspected organism. Antibiotic spectrum will often have to be broadened according to the severity of infection.

1.5.3 Management of preeclampsia/eclampsia/HELLP syndrome

Management of these syndromes is usually supportive and revolves around blood pressure control, use of magnesium sulphate to prevent seizures and timing of delivery. There are various guidelines proposed by different obstetric societies around the globe in regards to management. Of interest however are the emerging concepts on its long term cardiovascular and renal consequences (Mc Donald et al, 2008). Similarly acute fatty liver of pregnancy (AFLP) also demands supportive care and prompt delivery. Thrombotic thrombocytopenic purpura; which creates a diagnostic dilemma together with HELLP and AFLP is managed using plasma exchange. Studies have shown significant improvement in maternal mortality rates since its introduction (Martin et al, 2008).

1.5.4 Renal replacement therapy in pregnancy

When renal replacement therapy is indicated for medically not amenable acute complications like hyperkalaemia, fluid overload, metabolic acidosis, and uremic encephalopathy either of the modalities (haemodialysis; HD or peritoneal dialysis; PD) can be used during pregnancy however there are no head to head trials comparing the benefit of one over the other. However, studies do suggest that PD may interfere with utero-placental blood flow (Bui et al, 2003).

1.6 Outcome of obstetric AKI

Attempts have been made to derive factors to predict mortality associated with AKI. In general, AKI associated mortality seems to be variably increasing with increasing age, greater degree of illness severity at presentation, presence of chronic kidney disease, need for organ support in form of mechanical ventilation, hypotension or need for inotrope support and so on (Waikar et al, 2008). Degree of change in serum creatinine and need for dialysis as well are associated with increased mortality rates. These estimates however have not been analysed specifically in the setting of pregnancy related AKI.

Table 5 summarizes maternal mortality rates and renal outcome in pregnant women with AKI from different studies. In our experience prolonged duration of oliguria is associated with increased rate of dialysis dependency. Most of pregnant women with acute kidney injury come from rural areas and did not have antenatal check up (Khanal et al, 2010; Ahmad et al, 2001; Hassan et al, 2009). Antenatal check up not only helps in creating awareness among the pregnant mothers to seek help from midwives, it also brings high risk cases to notice and increases the likelihood of referral to experts on time. Sepsis including post abortal sepsis has been found to be associated with severe consequences and poor maternal outcome even in modern days in developing countries. This is probably from poor handling techniques and emphasizes the importance of need to increase the number of trained personnel like midwives to conduct delivery. Late referral to the tertiary care centres and delays in actually reaching the centre due to lack of infrastructure all contribute to the poor outcome. Significant and progressive improvement in mortality rates over decades is evident in table 6. This study analysed the data on pregnancy related AKI over 37 years. Although a progressive decline over each decade can be easily noticed, complications like HUS were associated with adverse maternal outcome. Thus close monitoring of high risk cases, timely recognition of complication, and institution of appropriate management intervention on time are of utmost importance (Stratta, 1996). A review on acute renal failure in hypertensive pregnant women which was conducted over 12 years included 9600 women with hypertension. 31 of these women developed AKI, all were in the postpartum period. Of these there were 2 maternal deaths and 50% of the patients from the pre-eclamptic group required dialysis. All patients had acute tubular necrosis (ATN). In the chronic hypertensive group with super imposed pre-eclampsia, 42% required dialysis and 3 had cortical necrosis (Sibai et al, 1990).

Author	Year	Study Pop with AKI	Mortality (%)	Dialysis dependent	Partial renal recovery	Complete renal recovery
Knapp	1957	23/32000 deliveries	48	-	-	-
Smith	1965	70	32	-	-	-
Chugh	1976	72	55.6	-	-	-
Prakash	1995	59	27	-	-	-
Stratta	1996	84	31	7	-	-
Kilari	2006	41	24.39	-	4	21
Hassan	2009	43	16.2	6	12	18
Khalil	2009	60	15	5	6	28
Khanal	2010	50	8	25	11	14
Prakash	2010	85	20	1	5	59
Arora	2010	57	28.1	3	5	24
Erdemoglu	2010	75	10.6	33.3% (required dialysis)		
Sivakumar	2011	59	23.72	-	10.16	54.23

Table 5. Renal outcome in Obstetric AKI.

Years	1958- 1967	1968- 1977	1978- 1987	1988- 1994
ARF (AKI)	60	298	535	562
PR-ARF	26(43%)	40(13.4%)	15(2.8%)	3(0.5%)

Table 6. Total Number and Main Causes of PR_ARF (obstetric AKI) Observed in 37 Years at Department of Nephrology and Clinical Obstetrics Torino, Italy (P Stratta,1996).

Both ante partum or post partum haemorrhage can lead to pre renal azotemia. Haemorrhage due to abruptio placentae has been found to be associated with increased risk of irreversibility of renal function in some series due to the development of cortical necrosis (Turney et al, 1989; Sibai et al, 1993). It is unclear why BRCN occurs more frequently during pregnancy, but this complication has been associated with septic abortions, preeclampsia, abruptio placentae, postpartum accidents, and haemorrhage. Bilateral renal cortical necrosis has been frequently mentioned to be associated with irreversibility of the renal function (Turney et al, 1989).

Foetal outcome is also poor. Intra-uterine death and still birth has been reported as high as 30-70% (Ali et al, 2004; Prakash et al, 2007; Khanal et al, 2010). High incidence of foetal loss was associated with increased incidence of dialysis dependency in mothers. This could be owing to the increased severity of illness (Khanal et al, 2010). Perinatal mortality is significantly low in neonates born to pregnant mothers without AKI as compared to those who developed AKI during pregnancy (Gul et al, 2004).

With the implementation of MDG 5 in developing countries, maternal mortality rates owing to all of these complications will hopefully improve along with improvement in foetal outcome.

1.7 Future perspective of obstetric acute kidney injury

Evident from the history, it is certain that maternal mortality rates from complications that can occur in pregnancy can be improved. Efforts have been put forward to increase the skilled birth attendants to assist delivery. However difficulties associated with overall health system and physical infrastructure, political instability and high illiteracy rates etc. creates hindrance to smooth development and therefore difficulty in achieving goals in developing countries.

Increased incidence of preterm deliveries associated with preeclampsia and its adverse long term renal/ cardiovascular outcome demand further research to understand the basis of the problem.

1.8 Recommendations

American college of obstetricians and gynaecologist guidelines
Society of Obstetric Medicine of Australia and New Zealand guidelines
Royal college of obstetricians and gynaecologists guidelines
WHO Guidelines on reproductive and sexual health

2. References

Agida ET, Adeka BI, Jibril KA: Pregnancy outcome in eclamptics at the University of Abuja Teaching Hospital, Gwagwalada, Abuja: a 3 year review. *Niger J Clin Pract*; 13: 394-398.

Ahmad W, Ziaulllah, Rizwanul-Haque M, Shari T. Acute renal failure: causes and outcome. *Proceeding Shaikh Zayed Postgrad Med Inst* 2001; 15:23-8.

Ahman E, Shah I: Unsafe abortion: worldwide estimates for 2000. *Reprod Health Matters* 2002; 10: 13-17.

Ali A, Zaffar S, Mehmood A, Nisar A. Obstetrical acute renal failure from Frontier Province: a 3 years prospective study. *J Postgrad Med Inst* 2004; 18:109-17.

Babinard J, Roberts P. Maternal and Child Mortality Development Goals: What Can the Transport Sector Do? *The International Bank for Reconstruction and Development/The World Bank*; 2006

Baylis C, Davison JM. Pregnancy and Renal Disease. In: Jurgen F, Johnson RJ, Feehally J. *Comprehensive clinical nephrology*. 4th ed. New York: Elsevier; 2010

Beaufils M. Pregnancy. In: Davison A, Cameron J, Grunfeld, Ponticelli C, Ritz E, Winearls C, Ypersele C. Oxford text book of clinical nephrology. 3rd ed. Great Clarendon Street: Oxford university press; 2005: 1604-12.

Bellomo R, Kellum J, Ronco C: Acute renal failure: time for consensus. *Intensive Care Med* 2001; 27: 1685-1688.

Bellomo R, May C, Wan L: Acute renal failure and sepsis. *N Engl J Med* 2004; 351: 2347-2349; author reply 2347-2349.

Bellomo R, Wan L, Langenberg C, Ishikawa K, May CN: Septic acute kidney injury: the glomerular arterioles. *Contrib Nephrol*; 174: 98-107.

Blantz RC: Pathophysiology of pre-renal azotemia. *Kidney Int* 1998; 53: 512-523.

Brown MA, Gallery ED: Volume homeostasis in normal pregnancy and pre-eclampsia: physiology and clinical implications. *Baillieres Clin Obstet Gynaecol* 1994; 8: 287-310.

Brown MA, Mangos GJ, Peek M, Plaat F: Renal Disease. In: Powrie R, Greene MF, Camann W. *de Swiet's Medical Disorders in Obstetric Practice.* 5th ed. Blackwell; 2010: 182-209.

Bui HT, Avjioglu E, Clarke A, Ellis D: Severe post-partum haemorrhage of the right kidney. *Aust N Z J Obstet Gynaecol* 2003; 43: 243-245.

Chugh KS, Singhal PC, Sharma BK, Pal Y, Mathew MT, Dhall K, et al.: Acute renal failure of obstetric origin. *Obstet Gynecol* 1976; 48: 642-646.

Cross S, Bell JS, Graham WJ: What you count is what you target: the implications of maternal death classification for tracking progress towards reducing maternal mortality in developing countries. *Bull World Health Organ*; 88: 147-153.

Davison JM, Dunlop W: Renal hemodynamics and tubular function normal human pregnancy. *Kidney Int* 1980; 18: 152-161.

de Bernis L, Dumont A, Bouillin D, Gueye A, Dompnier JP, Bouvier Colle MH (2000). Maternal morbidity and mortality in two different populations of Senegal: a prospective study (MOMA survey). *British journal of obstetrics and gynaecology*, 107(1): 68-74

Department of Reproductive Health and Research, World Health Organization. Unsafe abortion: global and regional estimates of the incidence of unsafe abortion and associated mortality in 2008. 6th Ed. 2011

Erdemoglu M, Kuyumcuoglu U, Kale A, Akdeniz N: Pregnancy-related acute renal failure in the southeast region of Turkey: analysis of 75 cases. *Clin Exp Obstet Gynecol*; 37: 148-149.

Ganesan C, Maynard SE: Acute kidney injury in pregnancy: the thrombotic microangiopathies. *J Nephrol*; 24: 554-563.

Goplani KR, Shah PR, Gera DN, Gumber M, Dabhi M, Feroz A, et al.: Pregnancy-related acute renal failure: A single-center experience. *Indian J Nephrol* 2008; 18: 17-21.

Gul A, Aslan H, Cebeci A, Polat I, Ulusoy S, Ceylan Y: Maternal and fetal outcomes in HELLP syndrome complicated with acute renal failure. *Ren Fail* 2004; 26: 557-562.

Hassan I, Junejo AM, Dawani ML: Etiology and outcome of acute renal failure in pregnancy. *J Coll Physicians Surg Pak* 2009; 19: 714-717.

Hill K, Abou-Zhar C, Wardlaw T (2001). Estimates of maternal mortality for 1995. *Bulletin of the World Health Organization*, 79(3): 182-193.

Hou HS. ARF in pregnancy. In: Molitoris BA, Finn WF. Acute renal failure: a companion to Brenner & Rector's The kidney. Philadelphia: W.B. Saunders; 2001: 304-11.

Hunt P, De Mesquita JB. Reducing maternal mortality: The contribution of the right to the highest attainable standard of health. University of Essex: 2010

Isler CM, Rinehart BK, Terrone DA, Martin RW, Magann EF, Martin JN, Jr.: Maternal mortality associated with HELLP (hemolysis, elevated liver enzymes, and low platelets) syndrome. *Am J Obstet Gynecol* 1999; 181: 924-928.

Jefferson A, Thurman JM, Schrier RW. Pathophysiology and Etiology of Acute Kidney Injury. In: Jurgen F, Johnson RJ, Feehally J. Comprehensive clinical nephrology. 4th ed. New York: Elsevier; 2010

Karumanchi SA, August P, Podymow T. Renal complications in normal pregnancy. In: Jurgen F, Johnson RJ, Feehally J. Comprehensive clinical nephrology. 4th ed. New York: Elsevier; 2010

Kennedy AC, Burton JA, Luke RG, Briggs JD, Lindsay RM, Allison ME, et al.: Factors affecting the prognosis in acute renal failure. A survey of 251 cases. *Q J Med* 1973; 42: 73-86.

Khalil MA, Azhar A, Anwar N, Aminullah, Najm ud D, Wali R: Aetiology, maternal and foetal outcome in 60 cases of obstetrical acute renal failure. *J Ayub Med Coll Abbottabad* 2009; 21: 46-49.

Khanal N, Ahmed E, Akhtar F: Factors predicting the outcome of acute renal failure in pregnancy. *J Coll Physicians Surg Pak*; 20: 599-603.

Khanna N, Nguyen H: Reversible acute renal failure in association with bilateral ureteral obstruction and hydronephrosis in pregnancy. *Am J Obstet Gynecol* 2001; 184: 239-240.

Kleinknecht D, Grunfeld JP, Gomez PC, Moreau JF, Garcia-Torres R: Diagnostic procedures and long-term prognosis in bilateral renal cortical necrosis. *Kidney Int* 1973; 4: 390-400.

Knapp RC, Hellman LM: Acute renal failure in pregnancy. *Am J Obstet Gynecol* 1959; 78: 570-577.

Krane NK: Acute renal failure in pregnancy. *Arch Intern Med* 1988; 148: 2347-2357.

Kribben A, Edelstein CL, Schrier RW: Pathophysiology of acute renal failure. *J Nephrol* 1999; 12 Suppl 2: S142-151.

Martin JN, Jr., Bailey AP, Rehberg JF, Owens MT, Keiser SD, May WL: Thrombotic thrombocytopenic purpura in 166 pregnancies: 1955-2006. *Am J Obstet Gynecol* 2008; 199: 98-104.

Maynard SE, Karumanchi SA, Thadhani R. Hypertension and kidney disease in pregnancy In: Brenner BM, Rector FC. The kidney. 7th ed. Philadelphia: W.B. Saunders; 2010: 1567-95

McCrae KR, Samuels P, Schreiber AD: Pregnancy-associated thrombocytopenia: pathogenesis and management. *Blood* 1992; 80: 2697-2714.

McDonald SD, Malinowski A, Zhou Q, Yusuf S, Devereaux PJ: Cardiovascular sequelae of preeclampsia/eclampsia: a systematic review and meta-analyses. *Am Heart J* 2008; 156: 918-930.

Najar MS, Shah AR, Wani IA, Reshi AR, Banday KA, Bhat MA, et al.: Pregnancy related acute kidney injury: A single center experience from the Kashmir Valley. *Indian J Nephrol* 2008; 18: 159-161.

Naqvi R, Akhtar F, Ahmed E, Shaikh R, Ahmed Z, Naqvi A, et al.: Acute renal failure of obstetrical origin during 1994 at one center. *Ren Fail* 1996; 18: 681-683.

Pertuiset N, Grunfeld JP: Acute renal failure in pregnancy. *Baillieres Clin Obstet Gynaecol* 1994; 8: 333-351.

Prakash J, Kumar H, Sinha DK, Kedalaya PG, Pandey LK, Srivastava PK, et al.: Acute renal failure in pregnancy in a developing country: twenty years of experience. *Ren Fail* 2006; 28: 309-313.

Prakash J, Niwas SS, Parekh A, Pandey LK, Sharatchandra L, Arora P, et al.: Acute kidney injury in late pregnancy in developing countries. *Ren Fail*; 32: 309-313.

Prakash J, Tripathi K, Pandey LK, Sahai S, Usha, Srivastava PK: Spectrum of renal cortical necrosis in acute renal failure in eastern India. *Postgrad Med J* 1995; 71: 208-210.

Prakash J, Vohra R, Wani IA, Murthy AS, Srivastva PK, Tripathi K, et al.: Decreasing incidence of renal cortical necrosis in patients with acute renal failure in developing countries: a single-centre experience of 22 years from Eastern India. *Nephrol Dial Transplant* 2007; 22: 1213-1217.

Ricci Z, Cruz DN, Ronco C: Classification and staging of acute kidney injury: beyond the RIFLE and AKIN criteria. *Nat Rev Nephrol*; 7: 201-208.

Robinson JJ, Wharrad H (2001). The relationship between attendance at birth and maternal mortality rates: an exploration of United Nations' data sets including the ratios of physicians and nurses to population, GNP per capita and female literacy. *Journal of advanced nursing*, 34(4): 445–455.

Royston E, Armstrong S (1989). *Preventing maternal deaths*. Geneva, World Health Organization

Scarpa RM, De Lisa A, Usai E: Diagnosis and treatment of ureteral calculi during pregnancy with rigid ureteroscopes. *J Urol* 1996; 155: 875-877.

Sibai BM, Ramadan MK. Acute renal failure in pregnancy complicated by hemolysis, elevated liver enzymes, and low platelets. Am J Obstet Gynecol 1993; 168 (6 pt 1): 1682-90.

Sibai BM, Villar MA, Mabie BC. Acute renal failure in hypertensive disorders of pregnancy. Pregnancy outcome and remote prognosis in thirty-one consecutive cases. Am J Obstet Gynecol 1990; 162 (3): 777-83.

Sivakumar V, Sivaramakrishna G, Sainaresh VV, Sriramnaveen P, Kishore CK, Rani Ch S, et al.: Pregnancy-related acute renal failure: a ten-year experience. *Saudi J Kidney Dis Transpl*; 22: 352-353.

Smith K, Browne JC, Shackman R, Wrong OM: Acute Renal Failure of Obstetric Origin: An Analysis of 70 Patients. *Lancet* 1965; 2: 351-354.

Stothers L, Lee LM: Renal colic in pregnancy. *J Urol* 1992; 148: 1383-1387.

Stratta P, Besso L, Canavese C, Grill A, Todros T, Benedetto C, et al.: Is pregnancy-related acute renal failure a disappearing clinical entity? *Ren Fail* 1996; 18: 575-584.

Strevens H, Wide-Swensson D, Hansen A, Horn T, Ingemarsson I, Larsen S, et al.: Glomerular endotheliosis in normal pregnancy and pre-eclampsia. *BJOG* 2003; 110: 831-836.

Uchino S, Kellum JA, Bellomo R, Doig GS, Morimatsu H, Morgera S, et al.: Acute renal failure in critically ill patients: a multinational, multicenter study. *JAMA* 2005; 294: 813-818.

Waikar SS, Liu KD, Chertow GM: Diagnosis, epidemiology and outcomes of acute kidney injury. *Clin J Am Soc Nephrol* 2008; 3: 844-861.

Weinstein L: Preeclampsia/eclampsia with hemolysis, elevated liver enzymes, and thrombocytopenia. *Obstet Gynecol* 1985; 66: 657-660.

World health organization. Population dynamics and reducing maternal mortality. 2009

URL:

http://www.who.int/making_pregnancy_safer/en/

http://www.somanz.org/pdfs/somanz_guidelines_2008.pdf

http://www.unfpa.org/public/publications/pid/4968

http://siteresources.worldbank.org/INTTRANSPORT/Resources/336291-1227561426235/5611053-1229359963828/tp12_maternal_health.pdf

Part 2

Polycystic Kidney Diseases

5

Extracellular Matrix Abnormalities in Polycystic Kidney Disease

Soundarapandian Vijayakumar
University of Rochester Medical Center,
Rochester, NY,
USA

1. Introduction

Polycystic kidneys diseases (PKD) are a group of monogenic kidney disorders that lead to cyst development in the kidneys. Polycystic kidney diseases are a common indication for renal transplantation and dialysis and a leading cause of end-stage renal disease (ESRD). There are two types of PKD, the autosomal dominant type called ADPKD with an estimated prevalence rate of 1:400-1:1000 worldwide (Torres & Harris, 2009) and autosomal recessive PKD (ARPKD) with an estimated prevalence rate of 1:10,000-1:20,000. ADPKD is the most common form of PKD, whereas ARPKD is the most lethal form and affects newborns. ADPKD is attributed to several mutations in one or both of the two genes PKD1 and PKD2, whereas ARPKD is attributed to mutations in the PKHD1 gene. The protein products of PKD1 and PKD2 are transmembrane proteins called polycystin 1 and polycystin 2 respectively, whereas the protein product of PKHD1, also a transmembrane protein is termed as fibrocystin. In ADPKD, the cysts arise throughout the nephron segments, whereas in ARPKD, cysts arise from the collecting duct as fusiform dilatations. In addition to kidney cysts, PKD patients generally also exhibit liver disease. Abnormalities in electrolyte secretion (Yamaguchi et al., 1997), EGF and cAMP dependent cell proliferation (Hanaoka and Guggino (2000); Richards et al., 1998), cell-matrix interaction (Ramasubbu et al., 1998; Wilson et al., 1992) and planar cell polarity (Fisher et al., 2006; Patel et al., 2008) have all been attributed to the disease mechanism of PKD. However, the exact cause of cystogenesis is yet unknown. Following Dr. Grantham's seminal work showing abnormal fluid secretion in ADPKD (Grantham, 1993), considerable progress has been done in that area (Magenheimer et al., 2006). Our understanding of the role of cAMP in cystogenesis has led to the development of high potency antagonists to vasopressin V2 receptors as therapeutic agents for ADPKD, which are currently undergoing clinical trials. There has been a great interest in understanding the role of primary cilia in PKD cystogenesis since several of the PKD associated proteins have been reported be localized to primary cilia in addition to other locations in the kidney epithelia (Yoder at al., 2002; Wang et al., 2007). However, the role of abnormal extracellular matrix in cystogenesis has not been pursued rigorously. This review will explore the current and past work that has been undertaken in this area.

2. Early observations of ECM abnormalities in PKD

The first observations of basement membrane abnormalities in PKD were observed as early as 1970 (Darmady et al., 1970). In 1980, Dr. Grantham and colleagues investigated 20 ADPKD cysts from five patients morphologically using electron microscope and observed that the basement membranes of PKD cysts were highly variable in appearance (Cuppage et al., 1980). Some were of reasonably normal thickness, whereas others were thickened or extensively laminated. Also, they observed that nearly every cyst had an abnormal basement membrane. In 1986, Patricia Wilson and her colleagues observed that human PKD epithelial cells in culture exhibited an extremely abnormal basement membrane morphology consisting of some banded collagen and numerous unique blebs or spheroids (Wilson et al., 1986). These blebs stained with ruthenium red, suggesting a proteoglycan component. After performing echocardiographic investigations on 160 ADPKD patients, 130 unaffected family members and 100 control subjects Hossack et al., concluded that cardiovascular abnormalities frequently accompanied PKD and suggested that PKD may be systemic disorder caused by abnormal extracellular matrix (Hossack et al., 1988). Using a murine model of congenital polycystic kidney disease, Ebihara et al., observed that that the components of the peri-cystic basement membrane appeared to diminish with time (Ebihara et al., 1988). Using mRNA measurements, they observed that in normal kidneys, mRNA levels for the B1 and B2 chains of laminin (currently the beta and gamma chains), were maximal at birth, and at 1 week for the alpha 1(IV) chain of collagen IV. With all three chains, the levels then rapidly declined. In contrast, mRNA for the collagen alpha 1(IV) chain in congenital polycystic kidneys was half normal 1 week after birth and then increased. Laminin B1 and B2 chain mRNAs were 80% of normal at 1 week but were maintained at that level. They concluded that there exists an abnormal regulation of basement membrane gene expression in congenital polycystic kidney disease. In 1992, Yashpal Kanwar and his colleagues observed altered synthesis and intracellular transport of proteoglycans by human ADPKD cyst derived epithelia (Jin et al., 1992). In a Kidney International article in 1993, Jim Calvet critically reviewed the question of whether the extracellular matrix abnormality is a primary defect in PKD (Calvet, 1993). Some early investigations suggested that tubular dilation could result from a loss of basement membrane tensile strength or to increased elasticity and that a tubular basement membrane was a primary defect in PKD. However, when basement membrane elasticity was measured directly by physical viscoelastic tests, it was determined that normal and cystic basement membranes were equally compliant. Jim Calvet also reviewed the results from two PKD model systems namely the *cpk* and *pcy* models. Primary epithelial cultures of *cpk* kidneys showed increased incorporation of ^{35S}methionine into collagen IV (approximately twofold) and into laminin. In human ADPKD kidneys, there is increased collagen IV mRNA level, particularly at end-stage. In the *pcy* mouse, laminin and collagen IV mRNA levels are somewhat increased in the early stages and more significantly elevated in the latter stages of the disease. Based on these results, it was suggested that a change in basement membrane collagen synthesis may not be a major factor in the initiation of cysts; the change is small and does not occur uniformly in early cyst formation. This review suggested that changes in ECM gene expression are more significant only at end-stage and therefore may be due to a late-stage compensatory response of the kidney to repair its tubular morphology.

3. Recent studies

In 2003, Joly et al., investigated nine ADPKD kidneys retrieved from patients with end-stage renal failure and one ADPKD kidney harvested before the onset of renal failure Joly et al., 2003). Using immunostaining, they showed that Laminin-332 and integrin β4 (a ligand of laminin-332) are aberrantly expressed in the pericystic ECM of ADPKD kidneys. Furthermore, using real-time PCR studies performed on the RNA extracted from primary cultures of the cystic epithelia derived from ADPKD kidneys as well as from PKD kidney tissues, they confirmed the abnormal expression of integrin β4 and laminin γ2 in ADPKD. The same authors presented a more rigorous study on the role of abnormal expression of laminin-332 in ADPKD cystogenesis (Joly et al., 2006). They demonstrated that ADPKD primary cultures synthesized and secreted laminin-332 which was then incorporated into the ECM of cysts that developed in matrigel cultures of these cells. Their studies also showed that addition of various amounts of laminin-332 in the 3D culture system enhanced cyst formation, as assessed by the number of cysts per optic field at day 7, whereas addition of laminin-332 function blocking antibody (D4B5) drastically reduced the number of cysts formed at day 7 by 73 ± 9%. Also, they showed that in monolayers, purified laminin-332 induced ERK activation and proliferation of ADPKD cells, and function-blocking anti-laminin γ2 antibody reduced the sustained ERK activation induced by epidermal growth factor stimulation. Using real time PCR, western blotting and immunostaining, we have demonstrated that laminin-332, particularly laminin γ2, is abnormally expressed in the PCK rat model of ARPKD (Vijayakumar et al., 2011). The abnormal expression of laminin-332 is not only observed in the cystic structures, but in the precystic collecting ducts also suggesting a possible role for aberrant laminin-332 expression in PKD cystogenesis.

A definitive role of ECM in PKD cystogenesis was established by Jeff Miner and his colleagues (Shannon et al., 1996). They generated a hypomorphic mutation in laminin α5, a major tubular and glomerular basement membrane component that is important for glomerulogenesis and ureteric bud branching by inserting a PGK*neo* cassette in an intron of the laminin α5 (*Lama5*) gene. *Lama5neo* represents a hypomorphic allele as a result of aberrant splicing. *Lama5neo/neo* mice exhibited PKD, proteinuria, and death from renal failure by 4 wk of age, whereas the mice that totally lack *Lama5* die *in utero* with multiple developmental defects. At 2d of age, *Lama5neo/neo* mice exhibited mild proteinuria and microscopic cystic transformation. By 2 wk, cysts were grossly apparent in cortex and medulla, involving both nephron and collecting duct segments. Tubular basement membranes seemed to form normally, and early cyst basement membranes showed normal ultrastructure but developed marked thickening as cysts enlarged. Overall, Laminin alpha5 protein levels were severely reduced as a result of mRNA frameshift caused by exon skipping. This was accompanied by aberrant accumulation of laminin-332 (laminin-5) in some cysts.

Recently, Ian Drummond and his colleagues have shown that in zebrafish, combined knockdown of the *PKD1* paralogs *pkd1a* and *pkd1b* resulted in dorsal axis curvature, hydrocephalus, cartilage and craniofacial defects, and pronephric cyst formation at low frequency (10-15%) (Mangos et al., 2010). Dorsal axis curvature was identical to the axis defects observed in *pkd2* knockdown embryos. Combined *pkd1a/b*, *pkd2* knockdown showed that these genes interact in axial morphogenesis. Dorsal axis curvature was linked to notochord collagen overexpression and could be reversed by knockdown of *col2a1* mRNA or chemical inhibition of collagen crosslinking. *pkd1a/b*- and *pkd2*-deficient embryos exhibited ectopic, persistent expression of multiple collagen mRNAs, suggesting a loss of negative feedback signaling that normally limits collagen gene expression. Knockdown of *pkd1a/b* also dramatically sensitized embryos to low doses of collagen-crosslinking inhibitors, implicating polycystins directly in the modulation of collagen expression or assembly. Embryos treated with PI3 kinase inhibitors wortmannin or LY-29400 also exhibited dysregulation of *col2a1* expression, implicating phosphoinositide 3-kinase (PI3K) in the negative feedback signaling pathway controlling matrix gene expression. They suggested that *pkd1a/b* and *pkd2* interact to regulate ECM secretion or assembly, and that altered matrix integrity may be a primary defect underlying ADPKD tissue pathologies.

Patricia Wilson and colleagues have recently implicated the role of focal adhesions in cystogenesis (Israeli et al., 2010). By comparing ARPKD cells, normal age matched human fetal (HFCT) cells and HFCT cells with 85% fibrocystin-1 silencing, they observed that fibrocystin-1-deficient cells had accelerated attachment and spreading on collagen matrix and decreased motility. Also, the fibrocystin-1-deficient cells were associated with longer paxillin-containing focal adhesions, more complex actin-cytoskeletal rearrangements, and increased levels of total β1-integrin, c-Src, and paxillin.

4. ECM and PKD fibrosis

One of the features of PKD, particularly ADPKD is the high variability in the age of onset of renal functional decline and the severity of disease progression. This variability has been attributed to mutations in other disease modifier genes (second hit) as well as epigenetic factors. Even if ECM abnormalities fail to be the primary PKD defect, it is almost certain that they play an important role in disease progression by contributing to renal fibrosis. Although there is not much known about the contribution of renal fibrosis in PKD disease progression, a recent review by Jill Norman presents a comprehensive and convincing argument to focus on this area of investigation (Norman, 2011). In this review, it is pointed out that in ADPKD, expansion of cysts and loss of renal function are associated with progressive fibrosis. Similar to the correlation between tubulointerstitial fibrosis and progression of chronic kidney disease (CKD), in ADPKD, fibrosis has been identified as the most significant manifestation associated with an increased rate of progression to ESRD. It is important to note that although fibrosis in CKD has been studied extensively, little is known about the mechanisms underlying PKD fibrosis. In this review, she concludes that the current data indicate that fibrosis associated with ADPKD shares at least some of the "classical" features of fibrosis in CKD (increased interstitial collagens, changes in MMPs, overexpression of TIMP-1, over-expression of PAI-1 and increased TGFβ) and points out that there are also some unique and stage-specific features. Based on the review of current literature, she suggests that epithelial changes appear to precede and to cause changes in the interstitium. It is also proposed that the development of fibrosis in ADPKD is a biphasic process with alterations in the cystic epithelia followed by changes in the interstitial fibroblasts and that reciprocal interaction between these cell types precipitate a progressive accumulation of ECM in the interstitial compartment. Since fibrosis is a major component of ADPKD it follows that preventing or slowing fibrosis should retard disease progression with obvious therapeutic benefits.

5. Conclusion

New studies cited in this review bring back the focus on the role ECM in PKD cystogenesis and fibrosis. Current results such as the study showing laminin alpha 5 hypomorphic mutation leads to cystic kidneys in mice, abnormal expression of laminin-332 in cysts and precystic tubules of PCK rat kidneys and aberrant expression of laminin-332 and integrin beta 4 in human ADPKD tissues, all point to the possible role of abnormal ECM in PKD cystogenesis. However it is possible that the mechanism that causes cyst formation is something other than the primary ECM defect and that the abnormal ECM observed in PKD aids in the progression of the disease by contributing to the mechanisms of fibrosis.

6. Acknowledgment

I thank the Department of Pediatrics, University of Rochester Medical Center for financial support and Prof. Vicente Torres, M.D., Ph.D. (Mayo Clinic) for his guidance and support.

7. References

Calvet JP. (1993) Polycystic kidney disease: primary extracellular matrix abnormality or defective cellular differentiation? Kidney Int. 43:101-108.

Cuppage FE, Huseman RA, Chapman A, Grantham JJ. (1980) Ultrastructure and function of cysts from human adult polycystic kidneys. Kidney Int. 17(3):372-81

Darmady EM, Offer J, Woodhouse MA. (1970) Toxic metabolic defect in polycystic disease of kidney: Evidence from microscopic studies. Lancet 1:547-550.

Ebihara I, Killen PD, Laurie GW, Huang T, Yamada Y, Martin GR, Brown KS. (1988) Altered mRNA expression of basement membrane components in a murine model of polycystic kidney disease. Lab Invest. 58:262-269

Fischer E, Legue E, Doyen A, Nato F, Nicolas JF, Torres V, Yaniv M, Pontoglio M. (2006) Defective planar cell polarity in polycystic kidney disease. Nat Genet. 38(1):21-3.

Grantham JJ. (1993) Homer Smith Award. Fluid secretion, cellular proliferation, and the pathogenesis of renal epithelial cysts. J Am Soc Nephrol. 3:1841-57.

Hanaoka K, and Guggino WB. (2000) cAMP regulates cell proliferation and cyst formation in autosomal polycystic kidney disease cells. J.Am. Soc.Nephrol.11:1179–1187.

Hossack KF, Leddy CL, Johnson AM, Schrier RW, Gabow PA. (1988) Echocardiographic findings in autosomal dominant polycystic kidney disease. N Engl J Med.319:907-12

Israeli S, Amsler K, Zheleznova N, Wilson PD. (2010) Abnormalities in focal adhesion complex formation, regulation, and function in human autosomal recessive polycystic kidney disease epithelial cells. Am J Physiol Cell Physiol. 298(4):C831-846

Jin H, Carone FA, Nakamura S, Liu ZZ, Kanwar YS. (1992) Altered synthesis and intracellular transport of proteoglycans by cyst-derived cells from human polycystic kidneys. J Am Soc Nephrol. 2:1726-33.

Joly D, Morel V, Hummel A, Ruello A, Nusbaum P, Patey N, Noël LH, Rousselle P, Knebelmann B. Beta4 integrin and laminin 5 are aberrantly expressed in polycystic kidney disease: role in increased cell adhesion and migration. Am J Pathol. 163:1791-800 (2003).

Joly D, Berissi S, Bertrand A, Strehl L, Patey N, Knebelmann B. (2006) Laminin 5 regulates polycystic kidney cell proliferation and cyst formation. J Biol Chem. 281:29181-29189.

Magenheimer BS, St John PL, Isom KS, Abrahamson DR, De Lisle RC, Wallace DP, Maser RL, Grantham JJ, Calvet JP. (2006) Early embryonic renal tubules of wild-type and polycystic kidney disease kidneys respond to cAMP stimulation with cystic fibrosis transmembrane conductance regulator/Na(+),K(+),2Cl(-) Co-transporter-dependent cystic dilation. J Am Soc Nephrol. 17:3424-37.

Mangos S, Lam PY, Zhao A, Liu Y, Mudumana S, Vasilyev A, Liu A, Drummond IA. (2010) The ADPKD genes pkd1a/b and pkd2 regulate extracellular matrix formation. Dis Model Mech.3(5-6):354-65.

Norman J. (2011) Fibrosis and progression of autosomal dominant polycystic kidney disease (ADPKD). Biochim Biophys Acta. 1812:1327-1336.

Patel V, Li L, Cobo-Stark P, Shao X, Somlo S, Lin F, Igarashi P. (2008) Acute kidney injury and aberrant planar cell polarity induce cyst formation in mice lacking renal cilia. Hum Mol Genet. 17:1578-90.

Ramasubbu K, Gretz N, Bachmann S. (1998) Increased epithelial cell proliferation and abnormal extracellular matrix in rat polycystic kidney disease. J Am Soc Nephrol. 9:937-45

Richards WG, Sweeney WE, Yoder BK, Wilkinson JE, Woychik RP and Avner ED. (1998) Epidermal growth factor receptor activity mediates renal cyst formation in polycystic kidney disease. J. Clin. Invest. 101:935–939

Shannon BM, Patton BL, Harvey, SJ and Miner JH. (2006) A Hypomorphic Mutation in the Mouse Laminin α5 Gene Causes Polycystic Kidney Disease. J Am Soc Nephrol 17: 1913–1922.

Torres VE and Harris PC. (2009) Autosomal dominant polycystic kidney disease: the last 3 years. Kidney Int.76(2):149-68.

Vijayakumar S, Parkhi K, and Stolar J. Abnormal expression and assembly of laminin-332 and laminin-511 in ARPKD. *JASN* 22: Kidney week 2011 abstracts, 576A-577A, (2011)

Wang S, Zhang J, Nauli SM, Li X, Starremans PG, Luo Y, Roberts KA, Zhou J. (2007) Fibrocystin/polyductin, found in the same protein complex with polycystin-2, regulates calcium responses in kidney epithelia. Mol Cell Biol. 27(8):3241-52.

Wilson PD, Schrier RW, Breckon RD, Gabow PA. (1986) A new method for studying human polycystic kidney disease epithelia in culture. Kidney Int. 30(3):371-8.

Wilson PD, Hreniuk D, Gabow PA. (1992) Abnormal extracellular matrix and excessive growth of human adult polycystic kidney disease epithelia. J Cell Physiol. 150:360-9.

Yamaguchi T, Nagao S, Kasahara M, Takahashi H, Grantham JJ. (1997) Renal accumulation and excretion of cyclic adenosine monophosphate in a murine model of slowly progressive polycystic kidney disease. Am J Kidney Dis. 30(5):703-709

Yoder BK, Hou X, Guay-Woodford LM. (2002) The polycystic kidney disease proteins, polycystin-1, polycystin-2, polaris, and cystin, are co-localized in renal cilia. J Am Soc Nephrol. 13(10):2508-2516

6

Angiogenesis and the Pathogenesis of Autosomal Dominant Polycystic Kidney Disease

Berenice Reed and Wei Wang
University of Colorado Anschutz Medical Campus, USA

1. Introduction

Occurring with an incidence between 1/400 - 1/1000 live births autosomal dominant polycystic kidney disease (ADPKD) is the most common potentially lethal genetic disorder affecting the kidney (Ecder et al., 2007). The disease results from mutation in either of two genes *PKD1,* located on chromosome 16p13.3 or *PKD2,* located on chromosome 4q21 and is inherited in an autosomal dominant manner (European Polycystic Kidney Disease Consortium, 1994; Mochizuki et al., 1996). The resulting disrupted expression of the respective encoded proteins polycystin 1(PC1) and polycystin 2(PC2) leads to development of multiple fluid filled cysts in the kidney. As the cysts continure to grow throughout life the normal kidney parenchyma is gradually lost and ensuing decrease of renal function occurs. ADPKD accounts for 4-10% of end-stage renal disease (ESRD) worldwide (Freedman et al., 2000; Konoshita et al., 1998). In 50% of cases loss of renal function, necessitating renal replacement therapy occurs by age 60 (Gabow et al., 1992). Renal cysts are often evident on ultrasound or magnetic resonance imaging (MRI) in children, who typically do not become symptomatic until reaching young adulthood (Chapman et al., 2003; Fick-Brosnahan et al., 2001; Seeman et al., 2003). While renal cysts are an invariable characteristic of ADPKD, cysts may also occur in other organs with differing degrees of severity. Hepatic cysts are found in 75% of patients with ADPKD by age 60, while pancreatic, arachnoid, seminal vesicle, and prostate cysts occur with a lower frequency (Ecder et al., 2007). ADPKD is a systemic disorder with abnormalities occuring in several organs and a significantly increased risk for cardiovascular complications among affected patients. The reader is referred to several comprehensive reviews on the clinical and and genetic determinants of ADPKD for more detailed description of disease attributes (Chapin & Caplan, 2010; Ecder et al., 2007; Pei, 2011).

The process of cystogenesis involves proliferation of the epithelial cells that line the kidney tubules. This process initially results in localized dilation of the tubule. Continued epithelial cell proliferation and fluid secretion into the cyst results in cyst growth, until the cyst pinches off from the tubule. While the development and growth of renal cysts is the key feature of this disorder, the exact mechanism and identity of the factors influencing this process remain to be determined. However, it is apparent that vascular changes including expansion and remodeling of the existing vascular network must occur in order to support the structural changes occurring in the ADPKD kidney. Accordingly, it is not surprising that cyst growth in ADPKD has been likened to growth of a benign tumor (Grantham & Calvet, 2001). Indeed, there are many similarities between tumor growth and cyst growth, both processes being marked by increased cell proliferation, changes in apoptosis, and angiogenesis. In this chapter we will focus on the process of angiogenesis, defined as the growth of new blood vessels by invasion and sprouting of the existing vessels, as distinct from embryonic vasculogenesis or de novo growth of blood vessels.

2. Angiogenesis

In order to understand the various signals and processes that define angiogenesis it is necessary to consider the main function of blood vessels, namely the supply of oxygen and nutrients to all the cells in the body. Much of our current knowledge of angiogenesis stems from studies of tumor biology. The fact that the diffusion limit of oxygen is approximately 100μm indicates that all blood vessels must be located within 100-200 μm of mammalian cells to ensure viability (Torres Filho et al., 1994). Subsequent studies by Judah Folkman et al. determined that tumor growth beyond 1-2-mm was angiogenesis dependent (Folkman, 2006). In health the endothelial cells that line the blood vessel lumen and the pericytes that surround the outer surface of the endothelial cells are in a "quiescent " state. This state is maintained by a balance of "pro" and anti-angiogenic growth factors that include vascular endothelial growth factor (VEGF), angiopoietin-1 (Ang-1), angiopoietin-2 (Ang-2), and various other chemokines and growth factors. Angiogenesis in the adult is defined by sprout formation or by splitting of a pre-existing blood vessel (Persson & Buschmann, 2011). The process of angiogenesis proceeds in several distinct stages and is initiated by a decrease in partial pressure of oxygen, which is detected by oxygen sensors on the endothelial cell. In the ADPKD kidney the growing cysts compress the renal vasculature resulting in decreased oxygenation. Hypoxia results in stabilization of the hypoxia-inducible factor (HIF-1). The HIF family, which in addition to HIF-1, also includes HIF-2 and HIF-3 are transcription factors. Structurally the HIF's comprise of a heterodimer of a regulatory α subunit and a constitutively expressed β subunit (Wang & Semenza, 1995). Angiogenesis is initiated by binding of HIF-1 to a hypoxia response element in the promoter of an angiogenic growth factor such as VEGF as reviewed by Hoeben et al. (Hoeben et al., 2004). In the case of new vascular sprout formation, when an angiogenic signal is detected by a quiescent blood vessel, the pericytes detach from the blood vessel wall and from the basement membrane. This is mediated by metalloproteinase (MMP) induced proteolytic degradation (Persson & Buschmann, 2011). Endothelial cells undergo several changes, loosening their cell junctions and allowing dilation of the vessel. VEGF increases endothelial cell permeability allowing escape of plasma proteins and formation of a provisional extracellular matrix (ECM). Endothelial cells next migrate onto the ECM surface mediated by integrin. Degradation of the ECM by proteases releases additional angiogenic growth factors from the ECM providing an angiogenic gradient that mediates migration and proliferation of the endothelial cells. One endothelial cell called a "tip cell" is instrumental in leading the migration, ECM degradation and consequent direction of growth of the vascular sprout. Maturation of the vessel requires return of the endothelial cells to a quiescent state, pericytes to attach and cover the vessel and down regulation of proteases by expression of tissue inhibitors of metalloproteinases (TIMP's). These changes are mediated by downregulated expression of VEGF and increased levels of Ang-1, transforming growth factor β (TGF-β), and platelet derived growth factor (PDGF) (Chung et al., 2010).

3. Angiogenic growth factors

In this section we will describe some of the most important angiogenic growth factors and their respective receptors with emphasis on the role of VEGF, Ang-1, and Ang-2 in the kidney in health and disease.

3.1 Vascular Endothelial Growth Factor (VEGF)

VEGF is a central mediator of angiogenesis inducing endothelial cell proliferation, sprouting and promoting vascular leakiness (Otrock et al., 2007). The VEGF family includes VEGF A, VEGF B, VEGF C, VEGF D and placenta growth factor (PIGF) each coded by a separate gene (Table 1).

Family Member	Receptor	Action
VEGF A	VEGFR-1/Flt-1 and VEGFR-2/Flk (with lower affinity)	Angiogenesis Endothelial cell migration Mitosis Permeability Chemotactic for macrophages and granulocytes
VEGF B	VEGFR-1/Flt-1	Embryonic angiogenesis
VEGF C	VEGFR-3/Flt-4	Mitosis, Migration, Differentiation, Survival of lymphatic endothelial cells
VEGF D	VEGFR-3/Flt-4	Lymphatic vasculature around broniole in lung
PIGF	VEGFR-1	Vasculogenesis Angiogenesis in ischaemia, Inflammation, Wound healing, Cancer related angiogenesis

Table 1. Receptor affinity and actions of VEGF family members.

The gene encoding VEGF A comprises of eight exons which by differential splicing encodes seven transcript variants that give rise to isoforms of differing amino acid length, VEGF-A_{206}, VEGF-A_{189}, VEGF-A_{183}, VEGF-A_{165}, VEGF-A_{148}, VEGF-A_{145} and VEGF-A_{121} respectively (Bevan et al., 2008; Hoeben et al., 2004). A further variant VEGF-A_{110} is derived by proteolytic cleavage. The major circulating isoform VEGF-A_{165}, is also abundant in the extracellular matrix. The VEGF polypeptides are homodimers although heteodimeric forms of VEGF-A and PIGF have also been described (DiSalvo et al., 1995). The biological functions of VEGF are mediated by binding to the tyrosine kinase receptors, VEGF receptor-1/fms-like tyrosine kinase-1 (VEGFR-1/Flt1), VEGF receptor-2/fetal liver kinase-1 (VEGFR-2/Flk-1) and VEGF receptor-3/ fms-like tyrosine kinase-4 (VEGFR-3/Flt4) (Ortega et al., 1999). The various members of the VEGF family bind to different VEGF receptors as shown in Table 1. VEGF-A (also referred to as VEGF) is expressed by mural cells including vascular smooth muscle cells and pericytes. In addition, in the kidney VEGF is expressed by both glomerular epithelial cells (podocytes) and by tubular epithelial cells (Robert et al., 2000).

The VEGF receptors are expressed on vascular endothelial cells as well as on a range of non-endothelial cells including monocytes and macrophages in the case of VEGFR-1 (Koch et al., 2011). In the kidney, glomerular endothelial cells express VEGFR-1 and VEGFR-2 (Thomas et al., 2000). Expression of VEGF is upregulated in response to hypoxia through upregulation of HIF-1α transcription factors. In addition, VEGF activity is modulated by binding to heparin sulfate and through interaction with the co-receptors neuopilin 1 and neuropilin 2, although the molecular mechanisms involved at present remain unclear (Koch et al., 2011). Both animal and human studies have shown that VEGF is essential for vascular repair and maintenance of normal glomerular function in the kidney (Dumont et al., 1995; Kitamoto et al., 2001; Satchell et al., 2004; Sugimoto et al., 2003). However, over expression of VEGF is also associated with glomerular disease, indicating that maintenance of normal VEGF level is essential for renal function (Veron et al., 2010). Significantly, a link between cystogenesis and VEGF was demonstrated in an animal study showing that increased expression of VEGF in renal tubules resulted in cyst formation (Hakroush et al., 2009).

Several recent studies have supported a role for an imbalance of angiogenic growth factor levels in disease processes including tumor growth, diabetes, chronic kidney disease (CKD), and cardiovascular disease (Futrakul et al., 2008; Guo et al., 2009; Persson & Buschmann, 2011; Lim et al., 2005; Nadar et al., 2004; Nadar et al., 2005). Endothelial dysfunction is a feature of patients with ADPKD (Schrier, 2006). VEGF has been shown to play a crucial role in preservation of the microvasculature, promoting vascular proliferation and repair in experimental renal disease (Chade et al., 2006; Iliescu et al., 2009; Zhu et al., 2004). Increased plasma levels of the VEGF inhibitor, soluble VEGF receptor (sFlt1) were recently demonstrated in CKD patients supporting an imbalance of the VEGF pathway in CKD (Di Marco et al., 2009). Tubulointerstitial hypoxia and capillary rarefaction are common features of progressive renal disease. In a study of patients with progressive or stable proteinuric renal disease attenuated VEGF-A expression by proximal tubular cells, despite activation of the intracellular response signalling pathway, was shown to distinguish those patients with progressive disease (Rudnicki et al., 2009).

Patients with ADPKD are at an increased risk for development of left ventricular hypertrophy (LVH) which is a significant risk factor for sudden death (Chapman et al., 1997). Increased plasma VEGF levels have been demonstrated in patients with target organ damage, defined as stroke, previous myocardial infarction, angina, LVH, and mild renal failure (Nadar et al., 2005). Mice expressing a *vegf b* transgene develop cardiac hypertrophy, further indicating that VEGF may also play a potential role in cardiac pathology associated with ADPKD (Karpanen et al., 2008).

3.2 Angiopoietins

The members of the angiopoietin family including Ang-1, Ang-2 and Ang-4 together with their soluble Tie-2 (tyrosine kinase with immunoglobulin-like and EGF-like domains 2) receptor are endothelial cell regulators with a role in the remodeling/maturation phases of angiogenesis. In addition to expression in endothelial and vascular smooth muscle cells Ang1, Ang2 and Ang-4 are also expressed in kidney (Fiedler and Augustin, 2006; Yamakawa et al., 2004; Yuan et al., 1999). Ang-1 is a Tie-2 agonist while Ang-2 in the absence of VEGF inhibits Ang-1/Tie-2 signaling as reviewed by Fiedler et al. (Fiedler and Augustin, 2006). Conversely, under conditions of adequate VEGF, or under hypoxic conditions as may exist in and around the growing renal cysts, Ang-2 stimulates angiogenesis (Lobov et al.,

2002). The activity of Ang-4 is similar to Ang-1 as it is a Tie-2 agonist and is expressed in human kidney proximal tubule epithelial cells. Activation of Tie-2 results in a downstream activation of P13K-Akt in endothelial cells leading to a survival pathway and cell chemotaxis (Makinde and Agarwal, 2008).

The plasma level of Ang-2 is elevated in patients with diabetes and is associated with indices of endothelial damage and dysfunction (Lim et al., 2005). Likewise, abnormal levels of serum Ang-1 and Ang-2 in hypertension have been linked with target organ damage (Nadar et al., 2005), thus indicating a potential role for angiopoietins in exacerbation of the extrarenal complications associated with ADPKD including left ventricular hypertrophy (LVH). LVH is a major risk factor for cardiac arrhythmias, sudden death, heart failure and ischemic disease in ADPKD (Schrier, 2006). Prevention of LVH in ADPKD is consequently a key factor in patient management. The expression of Ang-1, Ang-2 and Ang-4 in different tissues including human kidney proximal tubule cells is regulated by various factors including hypoxia, VEGF, angiotensin II and estrogen (Ardelt et al., 2005; Kitayama et al., 2006, Yamakawa et al., 2004).

4. Similarities between tumor growth and cyst growth in ADPKD

The polycystin proteins PC1 and PC2 have been likened to tumor suppressors associated with many types of neoplasia (Grantham, 2001). Thus, when polycystin function is impaired as in ADPKD, cells revert to a more de-differentiated state marked by high proliferative capacity (Song et al., 2009). It has been recognized for many years that angiogenesis is necessary to support tumor growth (Folkman, 1971). Moreover, many non-neoplastic diseases including macular degeneration, arthritis and endometriosis are angiogenesis dependent (Folkman, 2006). Thus a facilitative role for angiogenesis in ADPKD cyst growth is suggested. Tumor cell expression of angiogenic growth factors including VEGF is mediated by hypoxia (Pugh and Ratcliffe, 2003). Central to the hypoxia response pathway are HIF-1 and 2. HIF-1α is targeted for destruction via the ubiquitin pathway regulated by Von Hippel Lindau (VHL) protein. Inactivation of VHL results in an increase of HIF-1α and VEGF level (Na et al., 2003). In progressive renal disease human proximal tubular epithelial cells demonstrate activation of intracellular hypoxia response pathways and VEGF signaling despite attenuated expression of VEGF-A (Rudnicki et al., 2009). Growth of renal cysts results in compression of the surrounding blood vessels. Significantly, an up-regulation of hypoxia-angiogenic pathways has been reported based on a systems biology approach in ADPKD (Song et al., 2009). A further key mediator of angiogenesis is the tumor suppressor gene phosphatase and tension homolog deleted on chromosome 10 (PTEN) which is frequently deficient or inactivated in human cancers (Mirohammadsadegh et al., 2006; Ohgaki & Kleihues, 2007; Tam et al., 2007). Activation of mammalian target of rapamycin (mTOR) is a feature of ADPKD and this pathway is regulated by PTEN (Boletta, 2009; Rosner et al., 2008; Shillingford et al., 2006). Thus the literature supports similarities between tumorigenesis and ADPKD and underscores a potential role for angiogenesis in ADPKD cyst growth.

5. Evidence for angiogenesis in ADPKD kidneys

Abnormalities of the renal vasculature in polycystic kidneys have long been recognized based on early angiographic studies of the kidney (Cornell, 1970, Ettinger et al., 1969) Bello-

Reuss et al. presented evidence of angiogenesis in human ADPKD kidneys based on angiographic studies (Bello-Reuss et al., 2001). These studies illustrated development of a well-defined vascular capsule around human renal cysts in ADPKD. Many morphological malformations were shown in the cyst wall vessels including presence of spiral, tortuous, and dilated vessels. This aberrant morphology is also typical in tumors further illustrating similarities between ADPKD cyst growth and growth of a benign tumor. A later study by the same group using corrosion cast studies of human ADPKD kidneys confirmed the occurrence of angiogenesis (Wei et al., 2006). This study also reported loss of the normal kidney vascular architecture in addition to evidence of microvascular regression. The pathological changes related to angiogenesis in ADPKD may also result in increased vascular permeability thus facilitating fluid secretion into cysts (Wei et al., 2006).

6. Angiogenic growth factors in ADPKD kidneys

Angiogenesis is mediated by a shift in the balance towards expression of pro-angiogenic growth factors with concomitant decrease in anti-angiogenic factors. VEGF expression by renal cystic tubular epithelial cells and VEGFR-2 expression in endothelial cells in the small capillaries surrounding the cysts was demonstrated by Bello-Reuss et al. (Bello-Reuss et al., 2001). This contrasts with normal adult kidney where only weak expression of VEGF and VEGFR-2 are present in the collecting duct and surrounding capillaries (Simon et al., 1995). The demonstration of MMP-2 and integrin $\alpha_v\beta_3$ on the endothelial surface of blood vessels in ADPKD kidneys by the same authors further affirms the presence of components necessary for angiogensis in ADPKD kidneys. Subsequent studies in a rat model of polycystic kidney disease demonstrated increased expression of VEGF in the kidneys and sera of the cystic animals compared to control animals (Tao et al., 2007). Similarly, increased expression of both VEGF receptors, VEGFR1 and VEGFR2 was demonstrated in renal tubular epithelial cells in the polycystic kidneys of these animals. We have also demonstrated expression of Ang-2 and the Tie-2 receptor by cyst lining epithelial cells of human polycystic kidneys as illustrated in Figure 1 (unpublished data).

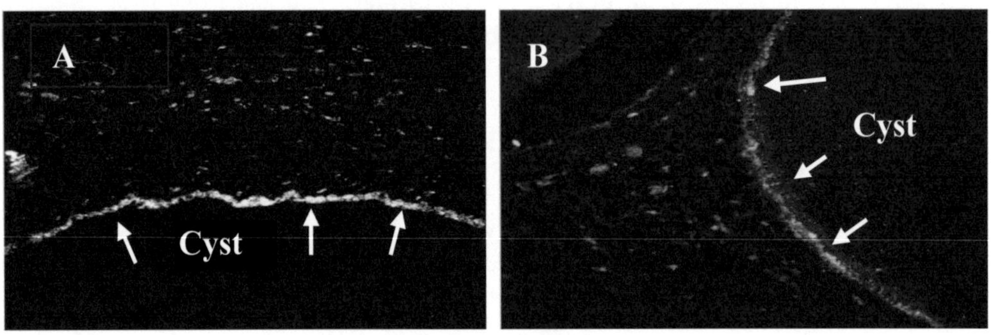

Fig. 1. Expression of Ang-2 (A) and Tie-2 (B) by ADPKD cyst lining cells. Arrows indicate cyst lining cells with Ang-2 staining shown by lighter shading in A and Tie-2 staining by lighter speckled shading in B.

These observations suggest a mechanism whereby secretion of pro-angiogenic growth factors by the cyst lining epithelial cells may result in stimulated growth of the blood vessels surrounding the cysts thus facilitating cyst growth as illustrated in Figure 2.

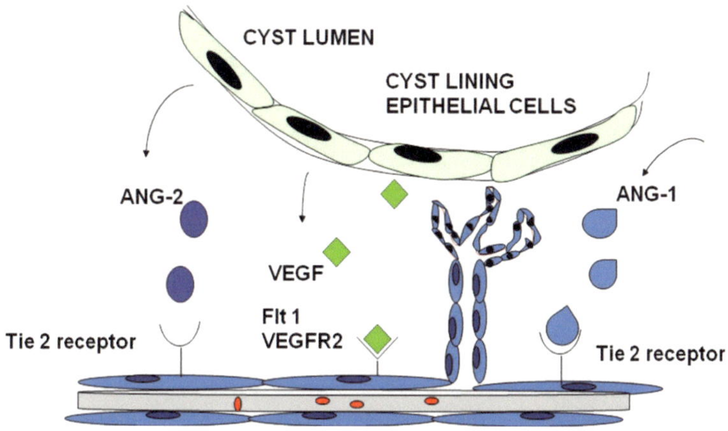

Fig. 2. Release of angiogenic growth factors by cyst lining and other cells in response to hypoxic stimulus stimulates angiogenesis.

However, the nature of renal injury in ADPKD is complex, apoptosis and loss of endothelium occurs which correlates with the severity of glomerular sclerosis and interstitial fibrosis (Wei et al., 2006). Thus both indication of angiogenesis and destabilization of the existing vasculature are apparent in ADPKD kidneys. This is supported by demonstration that changes in renal blood flow parallel increase in total kidney volume and precede decline in renal function measured by change in glomerular filtration rate (GFR) in ADPKD (Torres et al., 2007).

7. Angiogenic growth factors in ADPKD liver

Expression of angiogenic growth factors have also been demonstrated in cystic liver from human ADPKD patients and also in animal models of PKD.Upregulated expression of Ang-1, Ang-2 and their Tie-2 receptor has been demonstrated in the cholangiocytes that line hepatic cysts in ADPKD, supporting a role for angiogenic growth factors in liver cystogenesis (Fabris et al., 2006). Moreover, cyst fluid from hepatic cysts has been shown to contain VEGF (Amura et al., 2008; Nichols et al., 2004,). In a subsequent animal study factors secreted by liver cyst epithelia were shown to promote endothelial cell proliferation and development (Brodsky et al., 2009).

8. Serum levels of angiogenic growth factors are increased in ADPKD

We have previously reported that serum levels of VEGF and Ang-2 are elevated in children and young adults with ADPKD compared to age, sex, and renal function matched young subjects with diabetes as shown in Table 2 (Reed et al., 2011). In these children and young adults renal function was normal, mean eGFR 128 ml/min/1.73m^2. The level of VEGF detected in renal cyst fluid was comparable to the mean serum level. The plasma levels of the soluble VEGF receptor (sFlt1), an antagonist of VEGF, rise progressively with declining renal function in patients with CKD (Di Marco et al., 2009). The same study demonstrated an association between plasma sFlt1 level and endothelial dysfunction. In our own study we found that serum levels of sFlt1 ranged between <13-320 pg/ml in ADPKD patients, however normal healthy serum values were not available for comparison (unpublished data) (Table 2). It is important to note that both the circulating level of VEGF and level of the VEGF antagonist sFlt1 may play a role in implenting disease progression in ADPKD.

VEGF	**Mean± SD or range (N)**
Adult ADPKD patients (serum)	5910 ± 6188 pg/ml (N=46)
Children and young adults with ADPKD (serum)	2997 ± 5326 pg/ml (N=71)
Healthy adults (A) (serum) Healthy children (C) (serum)	249 ± 46 pg/ml (A) (Saito et al.,2009) 306 ± 39 pg/ml (C) (Heshmat & El Kerdany, 2007)
Urine adults with ADPKD	82.7-277.2 pg/ml (N =8) 183.9 - 469.2 ng/24h (N=8)
Renal cyst fluid	5940 ± 6757 pg/ml (N=5)
Soluble VEGF Receptor 1 (sFlt1)	
Adult ADPKD patients (serum)	93.8 ± 63 pg/ml (N =38)
Adult ADPKD patients (urine)	Not detected
Angiopoietin 1	
Adult ADPKD patients (serum)	37.54 ± 19.54 ng/ml (N=85)
Children and young adults with ADPKD (serum)	35.53 ± 21.03 ng/ml (N=71)
Healthy adults (A) (serum) Healthy children (C) (serum)	39.0 ± 9.9 ng/ml (A) (Park et al., 2009) 64.4 (23.5-101 ng/ml) (C) (Lovegrove et al., 2009)
Renal cyst fluid	None detected
Angiopoietin 2	
Adult ADPKD patients (serum)	3002 ± 1379 pg/ml (N=85)
Children and young adults with ADPKD (serum)	2352 ± 962 pg/ml (N=71)
Healthy adults (A) (serum) Healthy children (C) (serum)	1270 ± 494 pg/ml (A) (Park et al., 2007) 68 (68-1330 pg/ml) (C) (Lovegrove et al., 2009)
Renal cyst fluid	1657 ± 1035 pg/ml (N=5)

Table 2. Mean serum, urine or cyst fluid levels of angiogenic growth factors.

Several recent studies have supported a role for an imbalance of angiogenic growth factor levels in disease processes including tumor growth, diabetes, CKD and cardiovascular disease (Augustin et al. 2009; David et al., 2009; Lim et al., 2005; Nadar et al., 2004; Nadar et al., 2005). Endothelial dysfunction is a common feature of patients with CKD and VEGF has been shown to play a crucial role in preservation of the microvasculature promoting vascular proliferation and repair in experimental renal disease (Chade et al., 2006; Iliescu et al., 2009; Zhu et al., 2004). The plasma level of Ang-2 is elevated in patients with diabetes and is associated with indices of endothelial damage and dysfunction (Lim et al., 2005). Likewise, abnormal levels of serum Ang-1 and Ang-2 in hypertension have been linked with target organ damage (Nadar et al., 2005), thus indicating a potential role for angiopoietins in exacerbation of the extrarenal complications of ADPKD, including LVH.

As the growing cysts in ADPKD kidneys result in compression of the vasculature with attendant ischaemia (Ecder et al., 2007) these conditions are conducive for upregulated angiopoietin expression. Furthermore, kidney expression of Ang-1 and Ang- 2 is known to be upregulated by angiotensin II in addition to hypoxia (Kitayama et al., 2006., Yamakawa et al., 2004). Thus, as activation of the renin-angiotensin-aldosterone system (RAAS) occurs early in ADPKD, this may increase angiopoietin production with further injurious effects on the kidney vasculature and cyst growth.

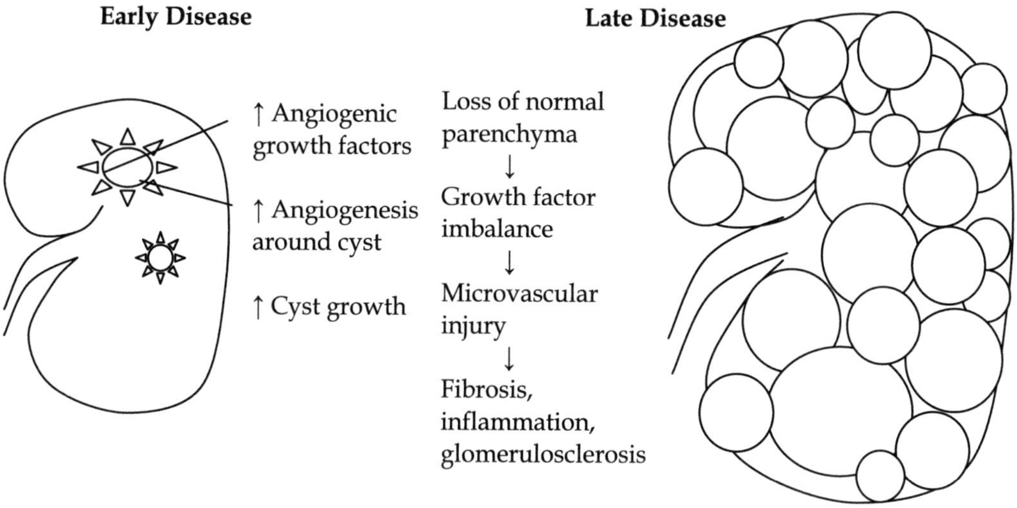

Fig. 3. Potential Role of Angiogenic Growth Factor in Renal Injury in ADPKD.

9. Serum levels of angiogenic growth factors correlate with renal and cardiac disease severity in ADPKD

Further evidence to support a role of angiogenic growth factors in the complications of ADPKD stems from our study in children and young adults (Reed et al., 2011). Measurement of VEGF, Ang-1 and Ang-2 in 71 children and young adults with ADPKD demonstrated strong correlations between $\log_{10}$ VEGF and both $\log_{10}$ total kidney volume and eGFR. (Table 3). In adult ADPKD patients no relationship between $\log_{10}$VEGF and total renal volume was found (N= 33). However, in adults there was a significant negative relationship between serum Ang-2 levels and eGFR (N = 85, p = 0. 04) that was not found in children and young adults. This indicates that VEGF may play a more significant role early in ADPKD, while Ang-2 may play a role in the progression of renal injury later in disease.

	Children			Adults		
IndependentVariable	**β**	**SE**	**P**	**β**	**SE**	**P**
	Dependent Variable					
	Log_{10} Total Renal Volume					
Log_{10} VEGF	0.0511	0.0183	0.0073			NS
Ang-1	0.0029	0.0014	0.0448	-0.00001	0.00001	NS
Ang-2			NS			NS
	eGFR					
Log_{10} VEGF	-0.0229	0.0080	0.0055	-0.0583	0.0307	0.06
Ang-1	-0.0010	0.0006	0.1058			NS
Ang-2			NS	-0.1380	0.0657	0.03

Table 3. Relationship of VEGF, Ang-1 and Ang-2 with renal structure and function.

We have demonstrated significant positive correlations between LVMI and Ang-1 and VEGF in young subjects with ADPKD as shown in table 4 (Reed, et al., 2011). The relationship between LVMI and serum VEGF was apparent even in the absence of overt hypertension. This is of particular relevance as patients with ADPKD are at an increased risk for left ventricular hypertrophy (LVH) (Chapman et al., 1997). Similarly, in 33 adults a near significant relationship between LVMI and Ang-1 was observed. No relationship between VEGF and LVM was apparent in adults. However, there was a significant relationship between Log_{10} Ang-1/Ang-2 and LVM. As Ang-2 has been reported to be both pro-angiogenic or promote vascular regression dependent upon the presence or absence of VEGF (Holash et al., 1999; Lobov et al., 2002) assessment of the Ang-1/Ang-2 ratio may be biologically relevant. Thus, angiogenic growth factor levels may help identify children at risk for cardiovascular complications. This is important because cardiac MRI and/or echocardiography are not routinely performed on young patients with ADPKD.

	Children			**Adults**		
Independent Variable	**β**	**SE**	**P**	**β**	**SE**	**P**
	Dependent Variable					
	LVM					
Log_{10} VEGF	0.0409	0.0078	<0.0001			NS
Ang-1	0.0014	0.0007	0.04	0.0004	0.0002	0.06
Log_{10} Ang-1/Ang-2			NS	12.2718	5.4447	0.03

Table 4. Relationship between VEGF, Ang1 and Ang-1/Ang-2 with Cardiac Structure.

10. Potential benefit of anti-angiogenic therapy in ADPKD

VEGF receptor inhibition by SU-5416 has been shown to significantly reduce liver cyst burden in pkd2(WS25/-)mice (Amura et al., 2007). Likewise, studies in the cy/+ rat model of polycystic kidney disease demonstrated that treatment with ribozymes to block VEGFR-1 and VEGFR-2 mRNA expression resulted in decreased cyst burden in the kidney (Tao et al., 2007). Metalloproteinase inhibition by batimastat in the cy/+ rat model has also been shown to significantly reduce kidney weight and cyst number in treated animals compared to untreated animals (Obermuller et al., 2001).

Several inhibitors that either target VEGF directly such as bevacizumab or those such as sorafenib and sunitinib that target receptor tyrosine kinases including VEGFR's and platelet derived growth factor receptors have shown some success in cancer therapy. Indicating that these drugs may have a potential role in ADPKD therapy. However, there are several side effects associated with both of these drug classes including but not limited to hemorrhage, decreased wound healing and hypertension. Side effects are a significant consideration in relation to ADPKD therapy where drug use must potentially be continued for life. While most anti-angiogenic drugs are targeted towards cancer therapy, bosutinib a receptor tyrosine kinase inhibitor targeting the Src/Abl kinases which also reduces VEGF activity is currently in phase II clinical trial for ADPKD (NCT01233869).

In terms of other anti-angiogenic targets, there are several ongoing cancer clinical trials with Ang-1 or Ang-2 inhibitors. Depending on the outcome of these ongoinig trials these drugs may hold some promise for future ADPKD therapy. It is also relevant that there are many naturally occurring inhibitors of angiogenesis including angiostatin, endostatin, vasostatin, TIMPs, thrombospondins, tumstatin, prolactin (inhibits both basic fibroblast growth factor and VEGF), vasohibin-1 and sFlt1 which may also have benefit in ADPKD. The therapeutic effects of several endogenous angiogenesis inhibitors including angiostatin, endostatin, tumstatin, vasohibin-1, and the synthetic derivative of bacterial cytogenin, 1-(8-hydroxy-6-methoxy-1-oxo-1H-2-benzopyran-3-yl) proprionic acid (NM-3) have been examined in animal models of diabetic nephropathy as reviewed by Maeshima and Makino (Maeshima & Makino, 2010). These angiogenesis inhibitors have been shown to reduce renal hypertrophy/hyperfiltration and reduce albuminuria when administered during the early stages of disease (Zhang et al., 2006, Ichinose et al., 2005, Yamamoto et al., 2004, Nasu et al., 2009, Ichinose et al., 2006). However, no human studies have been performed to date. In animal models of non-diabetic renal disease angiostatin treatment has resulted in both beneficial anti-inflammatory effects while the anti-angiogenic reduction in peritubular capillaries may worsen tubular hypoxia (Mu et al., 2009). Thus, with progressive renal diseases including ADPKD angiogenic growth factors may both promote renal injury or protect from hypoxia by maintenance of the peritubular capillaries. While in the early stages of ADPKD therapeutic restoration of normal angiogenic factor balance may be more beneficial, later disease stages may need a different approach to ameliorate increasing renal hypoxia. However, further research is necessary to explore the potential disparate roles of angiogenic growth factors in progression of ADPKD.

11. Conclusion

In this chapter we have presented evidence that angiogenesis may be an important factor in the pathogenesis of ADPKD. We have highlighted the similarities between cyst growth and growth of a benign tumour. Significantly, as has been demonstrated in other disease conditions circulating angiogenic growth factor levels are abnormally elevated even early in ADPKD and may indicate the severity of underlying renal and cardiac disease. Lastly, the benefits of anti-angiogenic therapies which target restoration of angiogenic growth factor balance remain to be determined in ADPKD but may hold future therapeutic promise.

12. Acknowledgment

This research was supported by Grant numbers M01RR00051, M01RR00069, the General Research Centers Program, National Center for Research Resources (NCRR/NIH; by NCRR/NIH Colorado CTSI Grant number UL1RR025780, by Grant DK34039 form NIH (NIDDK) and by the Zell Family Foundation. The content of this publication are the authors sole responsibility and do not necessarily represent the official NIH views.

13. References

Amura, C.R., Brodsky, K.S., Groff, R., Gattone, V.H., Voelkel, N.F. & Doctor, R.B. (2007) VEGF receptor inhibition blocks liver cyst growth in pkd2(WS25/-) mice. *Am. J. Physiol. Cell. Physiol.*, Vol.293, No.1, (July 2007) pp. C419-428, ISSN 0363-6143

Ardelt, A,A,, McCullough, L.D., Korach, K.S., Wang, M.M., Munzenmaier, D.H. & Hurn, P.D. (2005) Estradiol regulates angiopoietin-1 mRNA expression through estrogen receptor-alpha in a rodent experimental stroke model. *Stroke,* Vol.36, No.2, (February 2005), pp. 337-341, ISSN 0039-2499

Augustin, H.G., Koh, G.Y., Thurston, G. & Alitalo, K. (2009) Control of vascular morphogenesis and homeostasis through the angiopoietin-Tie system. *Nat. Rev. Mol. Cell. Biol.*, Vol.10, No.3, (March 2009), pp. 165-177, ISSN 1471-0072

Bello-Reuss, E., Holubec, K. & Rajaraman S. (2001). Angiogenesis in autosomal-dominant polycystic kidney disease. *Kidney Int.,* Vol. 60, No. 1, (July 2001), pp. 37-45, ISSN 0085-2538

Bevan, H.S., van den Akker, N.M., Qiu, Y., Polman, J.A., Foster, R.R., Yem, J., Nishikawa, A., Satchell, S.C., Harper, S.J., Gittenberger-de Groot, A.C. & Bates, D.O. (2008) The alternatively spliced anti-angiogenic family of VEGF isoforms VEGFxxxb in human kidney development. *Nephron Physiol.*, Vol.110, No.4, (November 2008),pp. 57-67, ISSN 1660-2137

Boletta, A. (2009) Emerging evidence of a link between polycystins and the mTOR pathways. *PathoGenetics,* Vol.2, No.1, October 2009, pp. 6, ISSN1755-8417

Brodsky, K.S., McWilliams, R.R., Amura, C.R., Barry, N.P. & Doctor, R.B. (2009) Liver cyst cytokines promote endothelial cell proliferation and development. *Exp. Biol. Med. (Maywood),* Vol.234, No.10 (October 2009), pp. 1155-1165, ISSN 1535-3702

Chade, A.R., Zhu, X., Mushin, O.P., Napoli, C., Lerman, A. & Lerman, L.O.(2006) Simvastatin promotes angiogenesis and prevents microvascular remodeling in chronic renal ischemia. *Faseb. J.*, Vol.20, No.10, (August 2006), pp. 1706-1708, ISSN 0892 6638

Chapin, H.C. & Caplan, M.J. (2010). The cell biology of polycystic kidney disease. *J. Cell Biol.*, Vol. 191, No. 4, (November 2010), pp. 701-710, ISSN 0021-9525

Chapman, A.B., Johnson, A.M., Rainguet, S., Hossack, K., Gabow, P. & Schrier, R.W. (1997) Left ventricular hypertrophy in autosomal dominant polycystic kidney disease. *J. Am. Soc. Nephrol.*, Vol.8, No.8, (August 1997), pp. 1292-1297, ISSN 1046-6673

Chapman. A.B., Guay-Woodford, L.M., Grantham, J.J., Torres, V.E., Bae, K.T., Baumgarten, D.A., Kenney, P.J., King, B.F., Jr., Glockner, J.F., Wetzel, L.H., Brummer, M.E., O'Neill, W.C., Robbin, M.L., Bennett, W.M., Klahr, S., Hirschman, G.H., Kimmel, P.L., Thompson, P.A. & Miller, J.P. (2003). Renal structure in early autosomal-dominant polycystic kidney disease (ADPKD): The Consortium for Radiologic Imaging Studies of Polycystic Kidney Disease (CRISP) cohort. *Kidney Int.,* Vol.64, No.3, (September 2003), pp. 1035-1045, ISSN 0085-2538

Chung, A.S., Lee, J. & Ferrera, N. (2010) Targeting the tumour vascalture: insights from physiological angiogenesis. *Nat. Cancer Rev.*, Vol.10, No.7, (July 2010), pp. 505-514, ISSN1474-175X

Cornell, S.H. (1970) Angiography in polycystic disease of the kidneys. *J.Urol.*, Vol.103, No.3, (July 1970), pp. 24-26, ISSN 0970-1591

David, S., Kumpers, P., Hellpap, J., Horn, R., Leitolf, H., Haller, H. & Kielstein, J.T. (2009) Angiopoietin 2 and cardiovascular disease in dialysis and kidney transplantation. *Am J Kidney Dis.,* Vol.53, No.5, (May 2009), pp. 770-778, ISSN 0272-6386

Di Marco, G.S., Reuter, S., Hillebrand, U., Amler, S., Konig, M., Larger, E., Oberleithner, H., Brand, E., Pavenstadt, H. & Brand, M. (2009) The soluble VEGF receptor sFlt1 contributes to endothelial dysfunction in CKD. *J. Am. Soc. Nephrol.,* Vol.20, No.10, (October 2009), pp. 2235-2245, ISSN 1046-6673

DiSalvo, J., Bayne, M.L.,Conn, G., Kwok, P.W., Trivedi, P.G., Soderman, D.D., Palisi, T.M., Sullivan, K.A., & Thomas, K.A. (1995) Purification and characterization of a naturally occurring vascular endothelial growth factor. Placenta growth factor heterodimer. *J.Biol.Chem.*, Vol.270, No.13, (March 1995), pp. 7717-7723, ISSN 0021-9258

Dumont, D.J., Fong, G.H., Puri, M.C., Gradwohl, G., Alitalo, K. & Breitman, M.L. (1995) Vascularization of the mouse embryo: a study of flk-1, tek, tie, and vascular endothelial growth factor expression during development. *Dev. Dyn.*, Vol.203, No.1, (May 1995), pp. 80-92, ISSN 1058-8388

Ecder, T., Fick-Brosnahan, G.M. & Schrier, R.W. (2007) Polycystic kidney disease, In: *Diseases of the Kidney*, eigth edition, R.W. Schrier, (Ed.), 502-539, Lippincott, Williams & Wilkins, ISBN 13:978-0-7817-9307-0, Philadelphia, PA., USA

Ettinger, A, Khahn, P.C. & Wise, H.M. (1969) The importance of selective renal angiography in the diagnosis of polycystic kidney disease. *J.Urol.*, Vol.102, No.2,(August 1969), pp. 156-161, ISSN 0970-1591

European Polycystic Kidney Disease Consortium. (1994). The polycystic kidney disease gene encodes a 14kb transcript and lies within a duplicated region of chromosome. 16. *Cell*, 77, pp. 881-894, ISSN 0092-8674

Fabris, L., Cadamuro, M., Fiorotto, R., Roskams, T., Spirli, C., Melero, S., Sonzogni, A., Joplin, R.E., Okolicsanyi, L. & Strazzabosco, M. (2006) Effects of angiogenic factor overexpression by human and rodent cholangiocytes in polycystic liver diseases. *Hepatology*, Vol.43, No.5, (May 2006), pp. 1001-1012, ISSN 1386-6346

Fick-Brosnahan, G,M,, Tran, Z.V., Johnson, A.M., Strain, J.D.& Gabow, P.A. (2001) Progression of autosomal-dominant polycystic kidney disease in children. *Kidney Int.*, Vol.59, No.5, (May 2001), pp. 1654-1662, ISSN 0085-2538

Fiedler, U. & Augustin HG. (2006) Angiopoietins: a link between angiogenesis and inflammation. *Trends Immunol.*, Vol.27, No.12, (December 2006) pp. 552-558, ISSN 0972-4567

Folkman, J. Tumor angiogenesis: therapeutic implications. (1971) *N Engl J Med.*,Vol.285, No. 21, (November 1971), pp. 1182-1186, ISSN 0028-4793

Folkman, J. (2006) Angiogenesis. *Ann Rev Med.*,Vol. 57, 1-18, ISSN 0066-4219

Freedman, B.I., Soucie, J.M., Chapman, A., Krisher, J. & McClellan, W.M. (2000). Racial variation in autosomal dominant polycystic kidney disease. *Am. J. Kidney Dis.*, Vol. 35, No.1, (January 2000) , pp. 35-39, ISSN 0272-6386

Futrakul, N., Butthep, P. & Futrakul, P. (2008) Altered vascular homeostasis in chronic kidney disease. *Clin. Hemorheol. Microcirc.*, Vol.38, No.3, (2008), pp. 201-207, ISSN (online) 1386-0291

Gabow, P.A., Johnson, A,M., Kaehny, W.D., Kimberling, W.J., Lezotte, D.C., Duley, I.T. & Jones, R.H. (1992). Factors affecting the progression of renal disease in autosomal-dominant polycystic kidney disease. *Kidney Int.*, Vol.41, No.6, (November 1992) pp. 1311-1319, ISSN 0085-2538

Grantham, J.J & Calvet J.P. (2001) Polycystic kidney disease: In danger of being X-rated? *Proc Natl Acad Sci U S A.*, Vol.98, No. 3, (January 2001), pp. 790-792, ISSN 0027-8424

Guo, Q., Carrero,J.J., Yu, X., Bárány, P., Qureshi, A.R., Eriksson, M., Anderstam, B., Chmielewski, M., Heimbürger, O., Stenvinkel, P., Lindholm, B. & Axelsson. J. (2009) Associations of VEGF and its receptors sVEGFR-1 and -2 with cardiovascular disease and survival in prevalent haemodialysis patients. *Nephrol. Dial. Transplant,* Vol.24, No.11, (November 2009), pp. 3468-3473, ISSN 0931-0509

Hakroush, S., Moeller, M.J., Thelig, F., Kaissling, B., Sijmonsma, T.P., Jugold, M., Akeson, A.L., Traykova-Brauch, M., Hosser, H., Hähnel, B., Koesters, R. & Kriz, W. (2009) Effects of increased renal tubular vascular endothelial growth factor (VEGF) on fibrosis, cyst formation, and glomerular disease. *Am. J. Pathol.,* Vol.175, No.5, (November 2009), pp. 1883-1895, ISSN 0002-9440

Heshmat, N.M. & El-Kerdany, T.H. (2007) Serum levels of vascular endothelial growth factor in children and adolescents with sytemic lupus erythematosus. *Pediatr. Allergy Immunol.,* Vol.18 No.4, (June 2007), pp. 346-353, ISSN 0905-6157

Hoeben, A., Landuyt, B., Highley, H.W., Van Oosterom, A.T. & DeBruijn, E.A. (2004) Vascular endothelial growth factor and angiogenesis. *Pharmacol. Rev.,* Vol.56, (December 2004,) pp. 549-580, ISSN 0031-6997

Holash, J., Maisonpierre, P.C., Compton, D., Boland, P., Alexander, C.R., Zagzag, D., Yancopoulos, G.D. & Wiegand, S.J. (1999) Vessel cooption, regression, and growth in tumors mediated by angiopoietins and VEGF. *Science,* Vol.284, No.5422, (June 1999(1994-1998, ISSN 0036-8075

Iliescu, R., Fernandez, S.R., Kelsen, S., Maric, C. & Chade, A.R (2009) Role of renal microcirculation in experimental renovascular disease. *Nephrol. Dial.Transplant.,* Vol. 25, No.4, (April 2004), pp.1079-1087, ISSN 0931-0509

Ichinose, K., Maeshima, Y., Yamamoto, Y., Kitayama, H., Takazawa, Y., Hirokoshi, K., Sugiyama, H., Yamasaki, Y. & Eguchi, K. (2005) Antiangiogenic endostatin peptide ameliorates renal alterations in the early stage of a type 1 diabetic nephropathy model. *Diabetes,* Vol.54, No.10, (October 2005), pp. 2891-2903, ISSN 0012-1797

Ichinose, K., Maeshima, Y., Yamamoto, Y., Kinomura, M., Hirokoshi, K., Kitayama, H., Takazawa, Y., Sugiyama, H., Yamasaki, Y. Agata, N, & Makino, H. (2006) 2-(8-hydroxy-6-methoxy-1-oxo-1h-2-benzopyran-3-yl) proprionic acid, an inhibitor of angiogenesis, ameliorates renal alterations in obese type 2 diabetic mice. *Diabetes,* Vol.55, No.5, (May 2006), pp. 1232-1242, ISSN 0012-1797

Karapanen, T, Bry, M., Ollila, H.M., Seppänen-Laasko, T, Liimatta, H., Kivelä, R., Helkamaa, T., Merentie, M., Jeltsch, M., Paavonen, K., Andersson, L.C., Mervaala, E., Hassinen, I.E., Ylä-Herttuala, S., Oresic, M., & Alitalo, K. (2008) Overexpression of vascular endothelial growth factor-B in mouse heart alters cardiac lipid metabolism and induces myocardial hypertrophy. *Circ.Res.,* Vol.103, No.9, (October 2008), pp. 1018-1026, ISSN 0009-7330

Kitamoto, Y., Takeya, M., Tokunaga, T. & Tomita,Y. (2001) Glomerular endothelial cells are maintained by vascular endothelial growth factor in the adult kidney. *Tohoku, J. Exp. Med.,* Vol.195, No.1, (September 2001), pp. 43-54, ISSN 0040-8727

Kitayama, H., Maeshima, Y., Takazawa, Y.,Yamamoto, Y., Wu, Y., Ichinose, K., Hirokoshi, K., Sugiyama, H., Yamasaki, Y. & Makino, H. (2006) Regulation of angiogenic factors in angiotensin II infusion model in association with tubulointerstitial injuries. *Am. J. Hyperens.,* Vol.19, No.7, (July 2006), pp. 718-727, ISSN 0895-7061

Koch, S., Tugues, S., LI, X., Gualandi, L. & Claesson-Welsh, L. (2011) Signal transduction by vascular endothelial growth factor receptors. *Biochem. J.,* Vol.437, No.2, (July 2011), pp. 169-183, ISSN 0939-4451

Konoshita, T., Okamoto, K., Koni, I. & Mabuchi, H. (1998). Clinical characteristics of polycystic kidney disease with end-stage renal disease. The Kanazawa Renal Disease Study Group. *Clin. Nephrol.,* Vol.50, No.2, (August 1998), pp. 113-117, ISSN 0301-0430

Lim, H.S., Lip, G.Y. & Blann, A.D. (2005) Angiopoietin-1 and angiopoietin-2 in diabetes mellitus: relationship to VEGF, glycaemic control, endothelial damage/dysfunction and atherosclerosis. *Atherosclerosis,* Vol.180, No.1 (May 2005) pp.113-118, ISSN

Lobov, I.B., Brooks, P.C. & Lang, R.A. (2002) Angiopoietin-2 displays VEGF-dependent modulation of capillary structure and endothelial cell survival in vivo. *Proc. Natl. Acad. Sci.,* Vol.99, No.17, (May 2002), pp. 11205-11210, ISSN 0027-8424

Lovegrove, F.E., Tangpukdee, N., Opoka, R.O., Lafferty, E.I., Rajwans, N., Hawkes, M., Krudsood, S., Looareesuwan, S., John, C.C., Liles, C. & Kain, K.C. (2009) Serum Angiopoietin-1 and -2 levels discriminate cerebral malaria from uncomplicated malaria and predict clinical outcome in African children. *PlosOne,* Vol.4, No.3, (March 2009), pp. e4912, ISSN 1932-6203

Maeshima, Y. & Makino, H. (2010) Angiogenesis and chronic kidney disease. Fibrogenesis and Tissue Repair, online Vol.3, No.13, (online August 5, 2010), ISSN 1755-1536

Makinde, T. & Agarwal, D.K. (2008) Intra and extravascular transmembrane signaling of angiopoietin-1-Tie-2 receptor in health and disease. *J. Cell. Med.,* Vol.12, No.3, (June 2008), pp. 810-828, ISSN 1582-1838

Mirmohammadsadegh, A., Marini, A., Nambiar, S., Hassan, M., Tannapfel, A., Ruzicka, T., & Hengge, U.R. (2006) Epigenetic silencing of the PTEN gene in melanoma. *Cancer Res,* Vol.66, No. 3, (July 2006) pp. 6546-6552, ISSN 0969-6970

Mochizuki, T., Wu, G., Hayashi, T., Xenophontos, S.L., Veldhuisen, B., Saris, J.J., Reynolds, D.M., Cai, Y., Gabow, P.A., Pierides, A., Kimberling, W.J., Breuning, M.H., Deltas, C.C., Peters, D.J. & Somlo, S. (1996) PKD2, a gene for polycystic kidney disease that encodes an integral membrane protein. *Science,* Vol.272, No.5266, (May 1996), pp. 1339-1342, ISSN 0036-8075

Mu, W., Long, D.A., Ouyang, X., Agarwal, A., Cruz, W.E., Roncal, C.A., Nakagawa, T., Yu, X., Hauswith, W.W. & Johnson, R.J. (2009) Angiostatin overexpression is associated with an improvement in chronic kidney injury by an anti-inflammatory mechanism. *Am. J. Physiol. Renal Physiol.,* Vol.296, No.1, (January 2009), pp. F145-F152, ISSN 0363-6127

Na, X., Wu, G,, Ryan, C.K., Schoen, S.R., di'Santagnese, P.A. & Messing, E.M. (2003) Overproduction of vascular endothelial growth factor related to von Hippel-Lindau tumor suppressor gene mutations and hypoxia-inducible factor-1 alpha expression in renal cell carcinomas. *J. Urol.,* Vol.170, No.2.pt1, (August 2003), pp. 588-592, ISSN 0970-1591

Nadar, S.K., Blann, A.D. & Lip, G.Y. (2004) Plasma and platelet-derived vascular endothelial growth factor and angiopoietin-1 in hypertension: effects of antihypertensive therapy. *J. Intern. Med.,* Vol.256, No.4, (October 2004), pp. 331-337, ISSN 0954-6820

Nadar, S.K., Blann, A., Beevers ,D.G. & Lip, G.Y. (2005) Abnormal angiopoietins 1&2, angiopoietin receptor Tie-2 and vascular endothelial growth factor levels in hypertension: relationship to target organ damage [a sub-study of the Anglo-Scandinavian Cardiac Outcomes Trial (ASCOT)]. *J Intern Med.,* Vol.258, No 4, (October 2005), pp. 336-343, ISSN 0954-6820

Nasu, T., Maeshima Y, Kinomura, M., Hirokoshi-Kawahara, K, Tanabe, K., Sugiyama, H., Sonoda, H., Sato, Y. & Makino, H. (2009) Vasohibin-1, a negative feedback regulator of angiogenesis, ameliorates renal alterations in a mouse model of diabetic nephropathy. *Diabetes*, Vol.58, No.10, (October 2009), pp. 2365-2375, ISSN 0012-1797

Nichols, M.T., Gidey, E., Matzakos, T., Dahl, R., Stiegmann, G., Shah, R.J., Grantham, J.J., Fitz, J.G. & Doctor, R.B. (2004) Secretion of cytokines and growth factors into autosomal dominant polycystic kidney disease liver cyst fluid. *Hepatology,* Vol.40, No.4, (October 2004), pp. 836-846, ISSN 1386-6346

Obermüller, N., Morente, N., Kränzlin, B., Gretz, N. & Witzgall, R. (2001) A possible role for metalloproteinaases in renal cyst development. *Am. J. Physiol. Renal Physiol.*, Vol. 280, No.3, (March 2001), pp. F540-F550, ISSN 0363-6127

Ohgaki, H. & Kleihues, P. (2007) Genetic pathways to primary and secondary glioblastoma. *Am. J. Pathol.,* Vol.170, No.5 (May 2007), pp. 1445-1453, ISSN 0002-9440

Ortega, N., Hutchings, H. & Plouët, J. (1999) Signal relays in the VEGF system. *Front. Biosci.*, Vol.4, (February 1999), pp. D141-D152, ISSN 1093-9946

Otrock, Z.K., Mahfouz, R.A., Makarem, J.A. & Shamseddine, A.I. (2007) Understanding the biology of angiogenesis: review of the most important molecular mechanisms. *Blood Cells Mol. Dis.,* Vol.39, No.2, (September-October 2007), pp. 212-220, ISSN 1079-9796

Park, J.H., Park, K.J., Kim, Y.S., Sheen, S.S., Lee, K.S., Lee, H.N., Oh, Y.J. & Heang, S.C. (2007) Serum angiopoietin-2 as a clinical marker for lung cancer. *Chest,* Vol.132, No.1, (July 2007), pp. 200-206, ISSN 0012-3692

Park, J., Choi, H., Kim, Y., Kim, Y., Sheen, S., Choi, J., Lee, H., Lee, K., Chung, W., Lee, S., Park, K., Hwang, S., Lee, K. & Park, K. (2009) Serum angiopoietin-1 as a prognostic marker in resected early stage lung cancer. *Lung Cancer,* Vol.66, No.1-2, (December 2009), pp. 359-364, ISSN 0169-5002

Pei, Y. (2011) Practical genetics for autosomal dominant polycystic kidney disease. *Nephron Clin. Pract.*, Vol.118, No.1, (January 2011), pp. c19-c30, ISSN 1660-8151

Persson, A.B. & Buschmann, I.R. (2011) Vascular growth in health and disease. *Front. Mol. Neurosci.*, Vol.14, Epub., August 2011, ISSN 0892-6638

Pugh, C.W. & Ratcliffe PJ. (2003) Regulation of angiogenesis by hypoxia: role of the HIF system. *Nat Med.* Vol.9, No.6, (June 2003), pp. 677-684, ISSN 1340-3443

Reed, B.Y., Masoumi, A., Elhassan, E., McFann, K., Cadnapaphornchai, M. & Schrier, R.W.(2011) Angiogenic growth factors in young patients with autosomal dominant polycystic kidney disease. *Am. J. Kidney Disease,* Vol.79, No.1, (January 2011), pp. 128-134, ISSN 0272-6386

Robert, B., Zhao, X. & Abrahamson, D.R. (2000) Coexpression of neuropilin-1, Flk1, and VEGF(164) in developing and mature mouse kidney glomeruli. Am. J. Physiol. Renal Physiol., Vol.279, No.2, (August 2000), pp. F275-282, ISSN 0363-6127

Rosner, M., Hanneder, M., Siegel, N., Valli, A., Fuchs, C. & Hengstschläger, M. (2008) The mTOR pathway and its role in human genetic diseases. *Mut. Res.*, Vol.659, No.3, (September - October), pp. 284-292, ISSN 1383-5718

Rudnicki, M., Perco, P., Enrich, J., Eder, S., Heininger, D., Bernthaler, A., Sarközi, R., Noppert, S.J., Schramek, H., Mayer, B., Oberbauer, R. & Mayer, G. (2009) *Lab. Invest.,* Vol.89, No.3, (January 2009), pp. 337-346, ISSN 0023-6837

Saito, T., Yamamoto, Y., Matsumura, T., Fujimura, H. & Shinno, S. (2009) Serum levels of vascular endothelial growth factor elevated in patients with muscular dystrophy. *Brain Dev.*, Vol.31, No.8, (September 2009), pp. 612-617, ISSN 0387-7604

Satchell, S.C., Anderson, K.L. & Mathieson, P.W. (2004) Angiopoietin 1 and vascular endothelial growth factor modulate human glomerular endothelial cell barrier properties. *J. Am. Soc. Nephrol.*, Vol.15, No.3, (March 2004), pp.566-574, ISSN1046-6673

Schrier, R.W. (2006) Optimal care of autosomal dominant polycystic kidney disease patients. *Nephrology* Vol.11, No.2, (April 2006), pp.124-130, ISSN 1320-5358

Seeman, T., Dusek, J., Vondrichova, H., Kyncl, M., John, U., Misselwitz, J. & Janda, J. (2003). Ambulatory blood pressure correlates with renal volume and number of renal cysts in children with autosomal dominant polycystic kidney disease. *Blood Press. Monit.*, Vol 8, No.3, (June 2003), pp. 107-110, ISSN 1359-5237

Shillingford, J.M., Murcia, N.S., Larson, C.H., Low, S.H., Hedgepeth, R., Brown, N., Flask, C.A., Novick, A.C., Goldfarb, D.A., Kramer-Zucker, A., Walz, G., Piontek, K.B., Germino, G.G. & Weimbs, T. (2006) The mTOR pathway is regulated by polycystin-1, and its inhibition reverses renal cystogenesis in polycystic kidney disease, *Proc. Natl. Acad. Sci. USA.*, Vol.103, No.14, (April 2006), pp. 5466-5471, ISSN 0027-8424

Simon, M., Grone, H.J., Johren, O., Kullmer, J., Plate, K.H., Risau, W. & Fuchs, E. (1995) Expression of vascular endothelial growth factor and its receptors in human renal ontogenesis and in adult kidney. *Am. J. Physiol. Renal Physiol.*, Vol.268, No.2 pt. 2, (February 1995), pp. F240-F250, ISSN 0363-6127

Song, X., DiGiovanni, V., He, N., Wang, K., Ingram, A., Rosenblum, N.D. & Pei, Y. (2009) Systems biology of autosomal dominant polycystic kidney disease (ADPKD): computational identification of gene expression pathways and integrated regulatory networks. *Hum. Mol. Genet.*, Vol.18, No.13, (July 2009), pp.2328-2343, ISSN 0964-6906

Sugimoto, H, Hamano, Y., Charytan, D., Cosgrove, D., Kieran, M., Sudhakar, A. & Kalluri, R. (2003) Neutralization of circulating vascular endothelial growth factor (VEGF) by anti-VEG antibodies and soluble VEGF receptor 1 (sFlt-1) induces proteinuria. *J. Biol. Chem.*, Vol.278, No.15, (April 2003), pp. 12605-12608, ISSN 0021-9258

Tam, K.F., Liu, V.W., Liu, S.S., Tsang, P.C., Cheung, A.N., Yip, A.M. & Ngan, H.Y. (2007) Methylation profile in benign, borderline and malignant ovarian tumors. *J. Cancer Res. Clin. Oncol.*, Vol.133, No.5, (May 2007), pp. 331-341, ISSN 0171-5216

Tao, Y., Kim, J., Yin, Y., Zafar, I., Falk, S., He, Z., Faubel, S., Schrier, R.W. & Edelstein, C.L. (2007) VEGF receptor inhibition slows the progression of polycycstic kidney diesease. *Kidney Int.*, Vol.72, No.11, (December 2007), pp.1358-1366, ISSN 0085-2538

Thomas, S., Vanuystel, J., Gruden, G., Rodríguez, V., Burt, D., Gnudi, L., Hartley, B.& Viberti, G. (2000) Vascular endothelial growth factor receptors in human mesangium in vitro and in glomerular disease. *J. Am. Soc.Nephrol.*, Vol.11, No.7, (July 2000), ISSN 1046-6673

Torres Filho I.P., Leunig, M.,Yuan, F., Intagletta, M. & Jain R.K. (1994) Noninvasive measurement of microvascular interstitial oxygen profiles in human tumor SCID mice. *Proc Natl Acad Sci U S A.*, Vol.91, No 6, (March 1994), pp. 2081-2085, ISSN 0027-8424

Torres, V.E., King, B.F., Chapman, A.B., Brummer, M.E., Bae, K.T., Glockner, J.F., Arya, K., Risk, D., Felmlee, J.P., Grantham, J,J., Guay-Woodford, L.M., Bennett, W.M., Klahr, S., Meyers, C.M., Zhang, X., Thompson, P.A.& Miller, J.P. (2007) Magnetic resonance measurements of renal blood flow and disease progression in autosomal dominant polycystic kidney disease. *Clin. J. Am. Soc. Nephrol.*, Vol.2, No.1, (January 2007), pp. 112-120, ISSN 1555-9041

Veron, D., Reidy, K.J., Bertuccio, C., Teichman, J., Villegas, G., Jimenez, J., Shen, W., Kopp, J.B., Thomas, D.B. & Turfo, A. (2010) Overexpression of VEGF-A in podocytes of adult mice causes glomerular disease. *Kidney Int.*, Vol.77, No.11, (June 2010), pp. 989-999, ISSN 0085-2538

Wang, G.L. & Semenza, G.L. (1995) Purification and characterization of hypoxia-inducible factor 1. *J. Biol. Chem.*, Vol. 270, No. 3, (January 1995), pp. 1230-1237, ISSN 0021-9258

Wei. W., Popov, V., Walocha, J.A., Wen, J., Bello-Reuss, E.(2006) Evidence of angiogenesis and microvascular regression in autosomal-dominant polycystic kidney disease kidneys: a corrosion cast study. *Kidney Int.*, Vol.70, No.7, (October 2006), 1261-1268, ISSN 0085-2538

Yamakawa, M., Liu, L.X., Belanger, A.J., AJ, Date, T., Kuriyama, T., Goldberg, M.A., Cheng, S,H., Gregory, R.J. & Jiang, C. (2004) Expression of angiopoietins in renal epithelial and clear cell carcinoma cells: regulation by hypoxia and participation in angiogenesis. *Am. J. Physiol. Renal Physiol.*, Vol.287, No.4, (October 2004), pp. F649-657, ISSN 0363-6127

Yamamoto, Y., Maeshima Y., Kitayama H., Kitamura S., Takazawa Y., Sugiyama H., Yamasaki Y. & Makino, H. (2004) Tumstatin peptide, an inhibitor of angiogenesis prevents glomerular hypertrophy in the early stage of diabetic nephropathy. *Diabetes*, Vol.53, No. 7, (July 2004), pp. 1831-1840, ISSN 0012-1797

Yuan, H.T., Suri, C., Yancopoulos, G.D. & Woolf, A.S. (1999) Expression of angiopoietin-1, angiopoietin-2 and the Tie-2 receptor tyrosine kinase during mouse kidney maturation. *J. Am. Soc. Nephrol.*, Vol.10, No.8, (August 1999), pp. 1722-1736, ISSN 1046-6673

Zhang, S.X., Wang, J.J., Lu, K., Mott, R., Longeras, R. & Ma, J.X. (2006) Therapeutic potential of angiostatin in diabetic nephropathy. *J. Am. Soc. Nephrol.*, Vol.17, No.2., (February 2006), pp. 475-486, ISSN 1046-6673

Zhu, X.Y., Chade, A.R., Rodriguez-Porcel, M., Bentley, M.D., Ritman, E.L., Lerman, A. & Lerman, L.O. (2004) Cortical microvascular remodeling in the stenotic kidney: role of increased oxidative stress. *Arterioscler. Thromb. Vasc. Biol.*, Vol. 24, No.10, (October 2004), pp. 1854-1859, ISSN 1079-5642

Part 3

The Renin-Angiotensin-Aldosterone Pathway

7

The Renin-Angiotensin-Aldosterone System in Dialysis Patients

Yoshiyuki Morishita* and Eiji Kusano
Division of Nephrology, Department of Medicine, Jichi Medical University, Tochigi, Japan

1. Introduction

Hypertension (HT) and cardiovascular disease (CVD) are common in dialysis-dependent chronic kidney disease (DD-CKD) patients. The renin-angiotensin-aldosterone system (RAAS) plays pivotal roles in the pathogenesis of HT in DD-CKD patients. Activated RAAS also increases inflammatory mediators, which was shown to be an independent predictor of CVD in DD-CKD patients. Recent meta-analyses suggested that antihypertensive pharmacotherapy may reduce CVD in DD-CKD patients. This review focuses on the physiological roles and blockade effects of RAAS for HT and CVD in DD-CKD patients.

2. The physiological roles of RAAS in DD-CKD patients

The role of RAAS in hypertensive DD-CKD patients was confirmed by the normalization of blood pressure (BP) upon administration of an angiotensin antagonist, saralasin. Normally, volume overload and elevation of BP result in suppression of RAAS production. Since this feedback is often incomplete in CKD patients, CKD patients often show HT and high or normal RAAS. Weidmann et al. reported that the renin levels of hypertensive hemodialysis-dependent CKD (HDD-CKD) patients were approximately twice as high as those of normal subjects. Parenchymal renal injury and renovascular disease may cause increased renin secretion in end-stage CKD. The prevalence of renal artery stenosis may be as high as 40% in patients starting HD, although the diagnosis was determined in only one-quarter of such a group before entering a dialysis program. Kimura et al. reported that plasma rennin activity (PRA) increased from 2.3±0.5 ng/ml/hr at just before initiation of HD to 6.5±1.3 ng/ml/hr over an 8- to 10-year period in HDD-CKD patients. These data suggested that renin secretion continued even after disuse atrophy of kidney with almost complete deterioration of its excretory function.

Activated RAAS increased inflammatory mediators, which is an independent risk factor for CVD. The mechanism is thought to be as follows. Activated RAAS directly increases pro-

* Corresponding Author

inflammatory gene expression and activates oxidative stress, leading to progressive inflammation of the vascular endothelium. In addition, among RAAS, mainly angiotensin II (AT II) stimulates vascular reactive oxygen species (ROS) production from sources such as NADPH oxidase and uncoupled endothelial nitric oxide (NO) synthesis. Increased ROS down-regulates NO activity that leads to endothelial dysfunction. AT II also directly increases pro-inflammatory gene expressions, such as VCAM-1 and MCP-1. Both processes lead to further recruitment of inflammatory cells and accelerate the vascular inflammatory response. On the other hand, the prognostic value of a high plasma aldosterone concentration (PAC) in HDD-CKD patients is unknown, where PAC is known to be associated with poor outcome in patients with cardiac disease. Kohagura et al. reported that lower PAC was independently predictive of death in hypertensive DD-CKD patients. The adjusted hazard ratio (95% confidence interval) of the lower PAC group was 2.905 (1.187–7.112, p=0.020). The significance of PAC became marginal when normalized with albumin or potassium. These results suggested that higher PAC was not associated with an increase in total and cardiovascular deaths among hypertensive HDD-CKD patients. The association between lower PAC and poor survival may be driven by volume retention and/or lower potassium level. Diskin et al. also reported that HDD-CKD patients with higher aldosterone levels tended to have longer survival.

Recently, it was found that RAAS components are expressed in many tissues, such as the heart, kidney, placenta, testis, eye, and lymphocytes. These local tissue RAAS components are suggested to contribute to tissue damage. Prorenin, which is a biosynthetic precursor of renin, is secreted not only by the kidney but also by many other tissues, whereas circulating renin is derived exclusively from juxta-glomerular cells of the kidney. Prorenin does not have enzymatic activity itself; however, several studies have reported that circulating prorenin could be taken up by tissues and contribute to activating local RAAS by binding (pro)renin receptor [(P)RR] and then that inactive prorenin is converted to the active form, which obtains enzymatic activity by conformational change. Recent studies have demonstrated that prorenin-(P)RR interaction activated tissue RAAS and contributed to the pathogenesis of organ damage in several diseases, such as HT and diabetes end organ damage; however, few studies have reported the role of tissue RAAS and prorenin in DD-CKD patients. Takemitsu et al. reported that arterial (P)RR may contribute to activate arterial tissue RAAS in HDD-CKD patients since arterial (P)RR mRNA expression was correlated with arterial angiotensin-converting enzyme (ACE) mRNA expression. Takemitsu et al. also reported that plasma prorenin concentration was correlated with PRA, plasma AT I level, plasma AT II level, and PAC level in HDD-CKD patients. Recently, we reported that the plasma prorenin level increased in HDD-CKD patients [147.1 +/- 118.9 pg/ml (standard value <100 pg/ml)]. The (P)RR mRNA expression level in peripheral mononuclear cells (PBMCs) also increased 1.41 +/- 0.39-fold in HDD-CKD patients compared with that in healthy control subjects ($p < 0.001$) (Figure 1). Plasma prorenin significantly correlated with plasma 8-hydroxydeoxyguanosine (8-OHdG) level ($r = 0.535$, $p < 0.001$), which is a useful marker for assessment of oxidative DNA damage in reactive oxygen species (ROS) including in HDD-CKD patients (Figure 2). These results suggested that tissue RAAS activated by circulating prorenin contributes to the regulation of plasma 8-OHdG level in HDD-CKD patients.

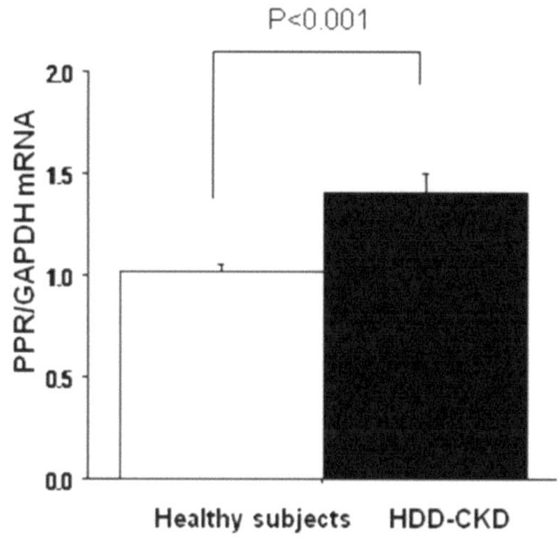

Fig. 1. (P)RR expression in peripheral blood mononuclear cells in healthy subjects (n=10) and HDD-CKD patients (n=49). Columns represent the mean ± s.e. (P)RR, prorenin receptor; HDD-CKD, hemodialysis-dependent chronic kidney disease (Morishita *et al.*, 2011).

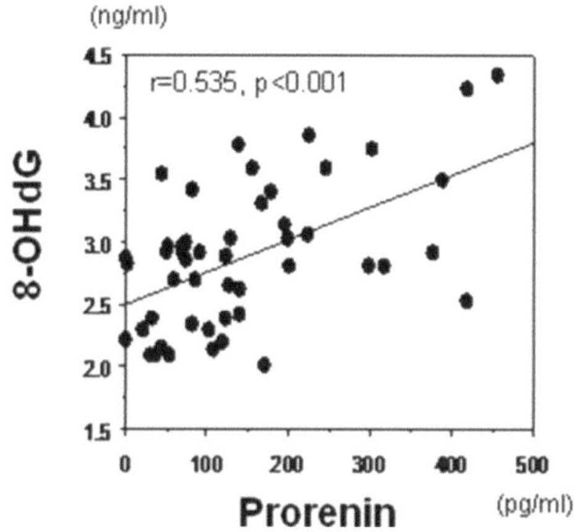

Fig. 2. Correlations of plasma prorenin level and 8-OHdG in hemodialysis-dependent chronic kidney disease patients. 8-OHdG, 8-hydroxydeoxyguanosine (Morishita *et al.*, 2011).

3. The blocked effect of RAAS in DD-CKD patients

3.1 HDD-CKD patients

Angiotensin-converting enzyme inhibitors in HDD-CKD patients

Tradolapril and captopril have been reported to be effective for HT in HDD-CKD patients. Zheng et al. reported that systolic BP (SBP) was decreased from 122.2±7.1 to 116.4±11.6 mmHg and diastolic BP (DBP) was decreased from 75.3±10.4 to 70.4±11.4 mmHg after 2-10 weeks by the administration of tradopril (2-8 mg/thrice a week (TIW)) after each HD session in 10 HDD-CKD patients. In that study, atenolol (25-50 mg/TIW) and/or amlodipine (10 mg/TIW) were also given if the patients had any member of these classes of drugs as part of their daily regimen. Wauterd et al. reported that captopril was administered orally in 2 daily doses of 25 to 200 mg in 8 HDD-CKD patients. These patients showed HT despite intensive ultrafiltration and conventional antihypertensive therapy. For 4 patients with the highest PRA, their BP was normalized by captopril alone. For the 4 remaining patients, captopril therapy was complemented by salt subtraction, which consisted of replacement of 1-2 liters of ultrafiltrate by an equal volume of 5% dextrose until BP was controlled. After an average treatment period of 5 months, BP of all 8 patients was reduced from 179/105 ± 6/3 (mean ±SEM) to 134/76 ± 7/5 mmHg (p <0.001) without a significant change in body weight. These clinical studies demonstrated that ACE inhibitor has beneficial effects to control BP in HDD-CKD patients. In addition, some studies reported that ACE inhibitors showed cardiovascular protective effects in HDD-CKD patients as follows. London et al. reported that perindopril (2-4 mg after each HD session) significantly reduced left ventricular mass (317±18 to 247±21 g, p=0.036) after 12 months in 14 HDD-CKD patients whereas a calcium channel antagonist, nitredipine (20-40 mg/day), did not when perindopril and nitredipine showed similar reductions of BP. Matsumoto et al. reported that imidapril (2.5 mg/day) significantly reduced left ventricular mass index (132±10 to 109±6 g/m^2, p<0.05) after 6 months; however, placebo did not produce a change in HDD-CKD patients. SBP and DBP were not significantly changed in either imidapril or placebo group. In that study, ACE was reduced (12±1 to 5±2 U/I, p<0.01) and PRA was increased (3.3±0.8 to 8.1±3.2 ng/ml/h, p<0.01) but plasma AT II and aldosterone (Ald) were not significantly changed (13±3 to 17±3 pg/ml and 365±125 to 312±132 pg/ml, respectively). These results suggested that the beneficial effect of imidapril against left ventricular mass was independent of BP lowering effect. Zannad et al. reported that no significant benefit was found with fosinopril (5-20 mg/day) for the prevention of cardiovascular events such as cardiovascular death, resuscitated death, nonfatal stroke, heart failure, myocardial infarction, or revascularization in HDD-CKD patients; however, there was a trend that fosinopril treatment may be associated with a lower risk of cardiovascular events after adjustment for risk factors. These lines of evidence suggested that ACE inhibitors are effective in controlling BP and preventing CVD in HDD-CKD patients. It is highly likely that the cardioprotective effects of ACE inhibitors are independent of their BP lowering effect in HDD-CKD patients.

Angiotensin receptor blockers in HDD-CKD patients

Saracho et al. reported on a multicenter, open 6 month study designed to test the tolerability and efficacy of losartan as an antihypertensive in 406 hypertensive HDD-CKD patients who were previously untreated, treated but uncontrolled, or treated with poor tolerability. There were significant reductions in pre- and postdialysis SBP and DBP at 3 months (pre SBP/DBP: 155 ± 15/84± 9 mmHg, post SBP/DBP: 140 ± 19/78± 10 mmHg) and 6 months (pre SBP/DBP: 152 ± 16/83± 9 mmHg, post SBP/DBP: 139± 18/77± 9 mm Hg) compared with those at baseline (pre SBP/DBP: 163 ± 16/88± 10 mmHg, post SBP/DBP: 148± 18/82± 9 mmHg). Shibasaki et al. reported that losartan (50 mg/day) reduced left ventricular mass index (-24.7±3.2%) after 6 months more than a calcium channel antagonist, amlodipine (5 mg/day: -10.5±5.2%), or an ACE inhibitor, enalapril (5 mg/day: -11.2±4.1%), although all three groups had similar decreases in mean BP. Kanno et al. reported that losartan (100 mg/TIW) reduced left ventricular hypertrophy (145±5 to 122±3 g/m^2, p<0.001) after 12 months in 24 diabetic patients on HD therapy whereas a placebo group showed no change. In this study, SBP and DBP were controlled below 140/90 mmHg with a calcium antagonist, benidipine (4-12 mg/day), and an α-blocker, doxazosin (2-4 mg/day). SPB was significantly decreased in both placebo and losartan groups after 12 months.These results suggested that this beneficial effect of losartan for left ventricular hypertrophy was independent of a BP lowering effect. Takahashi et al. stated that candesartan (4-8 mg/day) reduced cardiovascular events and mortality compared with placebo (16.3% vs. 45.9 and 0.0 vs. 18.9%, respectively) after 19.4±1.2 months in HDD-CKD patients in a stable condition and with no clinical evidence of cardiac disorder. In this study, the brain natriuretic peptide (BNP) level did not differ between the two groups at enrolment, whereas in patients who had not experienced a cardiovascular event at 12 months, the BNP levels were significantly increased in the control group but not in the candesartan group. Suzuki et al. reported that angiotensin receptor blockers (ARBs) (valsartan: 160 mg/day, candesartan: 12 mg/day, or losartan: 100 mg/day) treatment was independently associated with reduced cardiovascular events (hazard ratio, 0.51; 95% confidence interval, 0.33 to 0.79; p=0.002) compared with no ARB treatment group for 180 HDD-CKD patients in each group during a 3 year observation period. There were 34 (19%) fatal or nonfatal CVD events in the ARBs group and 59 (33%) in the no ARB group. BP did not differ between the ARBs group and the no ARB group during the observation period. After adjustment for age, sex, diabetes, and SBP, treatment with an ARB was independently associated with reduced fatal and nonfatal CVD events (hazard ratio, 0.51; 95% confidence interval, 0.33 to 0.79; p=0.002). These results demonstrated that ARBs are effective in controlling BP and preventing CVD in HDD-CKD patients. We predict that the cardioprotective effects of ARBs may be independent of their BP lowering effect in HDD-CKD patients.

Direct renin inhibitor

An oral direct renin inhibitor, aliskiren, is effective against essential HT by reducing PRA, resulting in suppression of RAAS; however, little was known about the effects of aliskiren in HDD-CKD patients. Recently, we reported on antihypertensive and potential cardiovascular protective effects of aliskiren, in hypertensive HDD-CKD patients. Aliskiren (150 mg/day) significantly reduced SBP and DBP after 2 month in hypertensive HDD-CKD patients (Figure 3). RAAS was suppressed by aliskiren treatment (PRA: 3.6±4.0 to 1.0 ±1.5 ng/ml/hr, p=0.004; AT I: 1704.0±2580.9 to 233. 7±181.0 pg/ml, p=0.009; AT II: 70.2±121.5 to 12.4±11.5 pg/ml, p=0.022) (Figure 4). Surrogate markers for cardiovascular disease such as BNP, high-sensitivity CRP (hs-CRP), and an oxidative stress marker, diacron-reactive oxygen metabolite (d-ROM), were inhibited by aliskiren (BNP: 362.5±262.1 to 300.0±232.0 pg/ml, p=0.043; hs-CRP: 6.2±8.1 to 3.5±3.7 mg/l, p=0.022; d-ROM: 367.0±89.8 to 328.3±70.9 U.CARR, p=0.022) (Figure 5). The levels of inhibition of these surrogate markers for CVD by aliskiren did not correlate with the decreased levels of BP. Two treatments were discontinued owing to an adverse event and symptomatic hypotension by aliskiren. The adverse event was eyebrow alopecia (1 patient). A possible connection of this event to aliskiren treatment could not be excluded. The symptomatic hypotension recovered to the basal level after aliskiren withdrawal. Increased serum potassium was not observed in any patients. Several studies reported that mean trough plasma aliskiren concentrations were increased by renal impairment; however, an increase in exposure did not correlate with the severity of renal impairment. Moreover, renal clearance of aliskiren was found to occur for only a small fraction (0.1-1.0%). These data suggest that adjustment of the aliskiren dose is unlikely to be required in HDD-CKD patients. Further studies will be required to investigate the pharmacokinetics of aliskiren in HDD-CKD patients. In summary, these results suggest that aliskiren is effective in BP control and extend the possibility that aliskiren may have cardiovascular protective effects in hypertensive HDD-CKD patients.

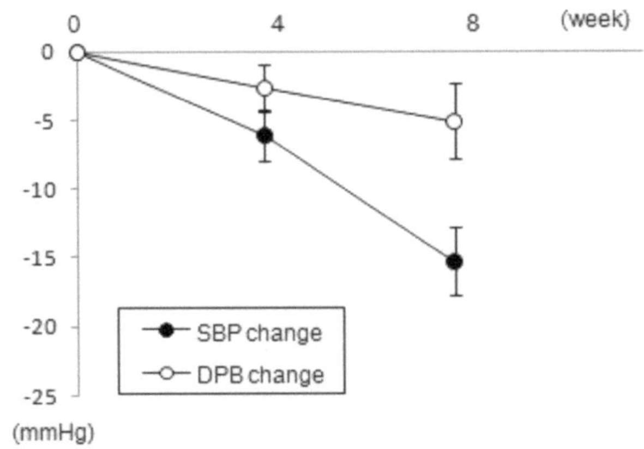

Fig. 3. Change in systolic blood pressure (SBP) and diastolic blood pressure (DBP) from baseline (Week 0) to Week 8 with aliskiren (150 mg/day) treatment in hemodialysis-dependent chronic kidney disease patients (Morishita *et al.*, 2011a).

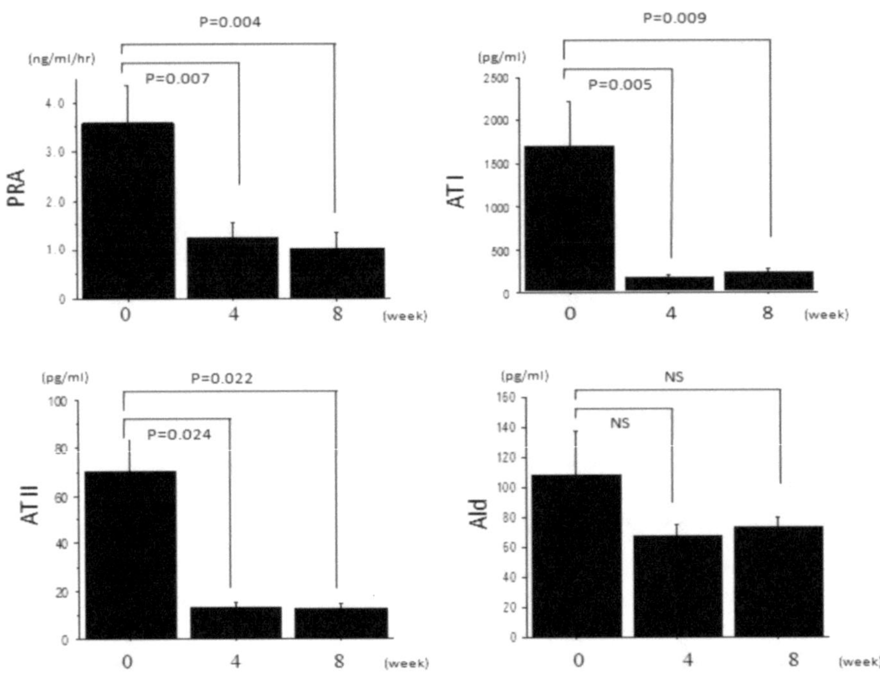

Fig. 4. Change in plasma renin activity (PRA), angiotensin I (ATI), angiotensin II (ATII), and aldosterone (Ald) by aliskiren treatment in hemodialysis-dependent chronic kidney disease patients (Morishita *et al.*, 2011a).

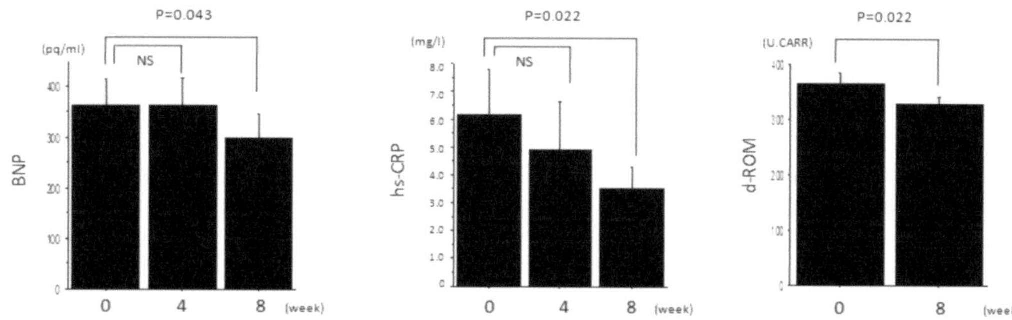

Fig. 5. Change in brain natriuretic peptide (BNP), highly sensitive C-reactive protein (hs-CRP), and diacron-reactive oxygen metabolite (d-ROM) by aliskiren treatment in hemodialysis-dependent chronic kidney disease patients (Morishita *et al.*, 2011a).

3.2 PDD-CKD patients

A few studies reported on a RAAS blockade effect in peritoneal dialysis-dependent CKD (PDD-CKD) patients. Fang et al. reported that a group (n=165) treated with ACE inhibitors/ ARBs had a significantly longer survival than an untreated group (n= 141) (log rank 19.191, $P < 0.001$) in PDD-CKD patients. After adjusting for age, BP, and other demographic and clinical parameters, multivariable Cox proportional hazards modeling showed that the use of ACE inhibitors/ARBs was associated with 62% reduced risk of death (HR 0.382, 95% CI 0.232-0.631, $P < 0.001$) in PDD-CKD patients. Jing et al. reported that ultrafiltration of a group treated with ACE inhibitors/ARBs group (n=38) had not changed after 12 months whereas that of an untreated group (n=28) had decreased ($P < 0.05$). The expressions of fibronectin, Transforming growth factor-β1 (TGF-β1) and vascular endothelial growth factor (VEGF) in dialysate effluent were significantly increased in the untreated group, but not in the group treated with ACE inhibitors/ARBs. These results suggested that RAAS blockade has beneficial effects for mortality and peritoneal function in PDD-CKD patients. Suzuki et al. reported that ARB (valsartan) slowed the decline in residual renal function independent of BP lowering effect in PDD-CKD patinets.

3.3 Caridioprotective effects of RAAS blockers independent of their BP lowering effect in DD-CKD patients

Increasing evidence suggested that elevation of RAAS contributes directly to cardiac hypertrophy via its growth factor properties on smooth muscle cells and cardiac myocytes among DD-CKD patients, independent of BP effects. RAAS also plays a role in cardiac fibrosis by stimulating TGF-β1 gene expression and induction of fibroblast proliferation and collagen deposition. RAAS blockers may directly effects for cardiac hypertrophy and fibrosis via these pathways independent of their BP lowering effects in DD-CKD patients. In addition, several studies reported that RAAS blockers showed beneficial effects for pulse wave velocity which is recognized as a potent predictor of mortality in DD-CKD patients, independent of their BP lowering effects. Further studies will be needed to investigate the mechanism of cardioprotective effects of RAAS blockade on DD-CKD patients.

3.4 Adverse effects of RAAS blockers in DD-CKD patients

ACE inhibitors showed several adverse effects in HDD-CKD patients. High-dose ACE inhibitors suppressed erythropoiesis and induced resistance to erythropoietin therapy in HDD-CKD patients. Occasionally, ACE inhibitors may cause anaphylactoid reactions with AN69 dialysis membrane in HDD-CKD patients by elevation of bradykinin level (Kammerl *et al.*, 2000). Hyperkalemia, which is a frequent concern in HDD-CKD patients independently of medication use, is the primary danger from RAAS blocking medications. Several clinical trials of ACE inhibitors, ARBs, and renin inhibitor in HDD-CKD patients tracked potassium levels. Increased hyperkalemia by these RAAS blockers in HDD-CKD patients was not observed in these trials. These results suggested that the risk of hyperkalemia by RAAS blocking is small.

4. Conclusion

From previous studies, it is suggested that RAAS blockade has a beneficial effect in controlling BP and preventing CVD in DD-CKD patients. However, the choice of the RAAS inhibitor as well as its use in the treatment of DD-CKD patients have to be carefully determined considering the possible adverse effects and potential interactions with other drugs being used in the treatment of DD-CKD patients. Further studies with an adequate sample size and a thorough design are still needed to determine the effect of RAAS blockade on DD-CKD patients.

5. Conflict of interest statement

None declared

Some parts of this manuscript were reported in Cardiovascular & Hematological Agents in Medical Chemistry (submitted), Hypertension Research (2011), 34, 308-313 and Clinical Experimental Nephrology(2011), 15, 398-404.

6. References

Agarwal, R., Nissenson, A.R., Batlle, D., Coyne, D.W., Trout, J.R., Warnock, D.G., 2003. Prevalence, treatment, and control of hypertension in chronic hemodialysis patients in the United States. Am J Med 115, 291-297.

Agarwal, R., Sinha, A.D., 2009. Cardiovascular protection with antihypertensive drugs in dialysis patients: systematic review and meta-analysis. Hypertension 53, 860-866.

Austin, E.W., Parrish, J.M., Kinder, D.H., Bull, R.J., 1996. Lipid peroxidation and formation of 8-hydroxydeoxyguanosine from acute doses of halogenated acetic acids. Fundam Appl Toxicol 31, 77-82.

Blankestijn, P.J., Ligtenberg, G., 2004. Volume-independent mechanisms of hypertension in hemodialysis patients: clinical implications. Semin Dial 17, 265-269.

Collins, A.J., Roberts, T.L., St Peter, W.L., Chen, S.C., Ebben, J., Constantini, E., 2002. United States Renal Data System assessment of the impact of the National Kidney Foundation-Dialysis Outcomes Quality Initiative guidelines. Am J Kidney Dis 39, 784-795.

Cooper, A.C., Robinson, G., Vinson, G.P., Cheung, W.T., Broughton Pipkin, F., 1999. The localization and expression of the renin-angiotensin system in the human placenta throughout pregnancy. Placenta 20, 467-474.

Crawford, D.C., Chobanian, A.V., Brecher, P., 1994. Angiotensin II induces fibronectin expression associated with cardiac fibrosis in the rat. Circ Res 74, 727-739.

Diskin, C.J., Stokes, T.J., Dansby, L.M., Carter, T.B., Radcliff, L., 2004. The clinical significance of aldosterone in ESRD: Part II. Nephrol Dial Transplant 19, 1331-1332; author reply 1332.

Dostal, D.E., Baker, K.M., 1999. The cardiac renin-angiotensin system: conceptual, or a regulator of cardiac function? Circ Res 85, 643-650.

Fang, W., Oreopoulos, D.G., Bargman, J.M., 2008. Use of ACE inhibitors or angiotensin receptor blockers and survival in patients on peritoneal dialysis. Nephrol Dial Transplant 23, 3704-3710.

Heerspink, H.J., Ninomiya, T., Zoungas, S., de Zeeuw, D., Grobbee, D.E., Jardine, M.J., Gallagher, M., Roberts, M.A., Cass, A., Neal, B., Perkovic, V., 2009. Effect of lowering blood pressure on cardiovascular events and mortality in patients on dialysis: a systematic review and meta-analysis of randomised controlled trials. Lancet 373, 1009-1015.

Herzog, C.A., Ma, J.Z., Collins, A.J., 2002. Long-term survival of dialysis patients in the United States with prosthetic heart valves: should ACC/AHA practice guidelines on valve selection be modified? Circulation 105, 1336-1341.

Hsueh, W.A., Baxter, J.D., 1991. Human prorenin. Hypertension 17, 469-477.

Huang, W.H., Hsu, C.W., Chen, Y.C., Hung, C.C., Huang, J.Y., Lin, J.L., Yang, C.W., 2007. Angiotensin II receptor antagonists supplementation is associated with arterial stiffness: insight from a retrospective study in 116 peritoneal dialysis patients. Ren Fail 29, 843-848.

Ichihara, A., Hayashi, M., Kaneshiro, Y., Suzuki, F., Nakagawa, T., Tada, Y., Koura, Y., Nishiyama, A., Okada, H., Uddin, M.N., Nabi, A.H., Ishida, Y., Inagami, T., Saruta, T., 2004. Inhibition of diabetic nephropathy by a decoy peptide corresponding to the "handle" region for nonproteolytic activation of prorenin. J Clin Invest 114, 1128-1135.

Ichihara, A., Hayashi, M., Kaneshiro, Y., Takemitsu, T., Homma, K., Kanno, Y., Yoshizawa, M., Furukawa, T., Takenaka, T., Saruta, T., 2005. Low doses of losartan and trandolapril improve arterial stiffness in hemodialysis patients. Am J Kidney Dis 45, 866-874.

Ichihara, A., Kaneshiro, Y., Takemitsu, T., Sakoda, M., Suzuki, F., Nakagawa, T., Nishiyama, A., Inagami, T., Hayashi, M., 2006. Nonproteolytic activation of prorenin contributes to development of cardiac fibrosis in genetic hypertension. Hypertension 47, 894-900.

Ito, S., Nakura, N., Le Breton, S., Keefe, D., 2010. Efficacy and safety of aliskiren in Japanese hypertensive patients with renal dysfunction. Hypertens Res 33, 62-66.

Jing, S., Kezhou, Y., Hong, Z., Qun, W., Rong, W., 2010. Effect of renin-angiotensin system inhibitors on prevention of peritoneal fibrosis in peritoneal dialysis patients. Nephrology (Carlton) 15, 27-32.

Jurewicz, M., McDermott, D.H., Sechler, J.M., Tinckam, K., Takakura, A., Carpenter, C.B., Milford, E., Abdi, R., 2007. Human T and natural killer cells possess a functional renin-angiotensin system: further mechanisms of angiotensin II-induced inflammation. J Am Soc Nephrol 18, 1093-1102.

Kammerl, M.C., Schaefer, R.M., Schweda, F., Schreiber, M., Riegger, G.A., Kramer, B.K., 2000. Extracorporal therapy with AN69 membranes in combination with ACE inhibition causing severe anaphylactoid reactions: still a current problem? Clin Nephrol 53, 486-488.

Kanno, Y., Kaneko, K., Kaneko, M., Kotaki, S., Mimura, T., Takane, H., Suzuki, H., 2004. Angiotensin receptor antagonist regresses left ventricular hypertrophy associated with diabetic nephropathy in dialysis patients. J Cardiovasc Pharmacol 43, 380-386.

Kimura, G., Takahashi, N., Kawano, Y., Inenaga, T., Inoue, T., Nakamura, S., Matsuoka, H., Omae, T., 1995. Plasma renin activity in hemodialyzed patients during long-term follow-up. Am J Kidney Dis 25, 589-592.

Kohagura, K., Higashiuesato, Y., Ishiki, T., Yoshi, S., Ohya, Y., Iseki, K., Takishita, S., 2006. Plasma aldosterone in hypertensive patients on chronic hemodialysis: distribution, determinants and impact on survival. Hypertens Res 29, 597-604.

Krop, M., Danser, A.H., 2008. Circulating versus tissue renin-angiotensin system: on the origin of (pro)renin. Curr Hypertens Rep 10, 112-118.

Kupfahl, C., Pink, D., Friedrich, K., Zurbrugg, H.R., Neuss, M., Warnecke, C., Fielitz, J., Graf, K., Fleck, E., Regitz-Zagrosek, V., 2000. Angiotensin II directly increases transforming growth factor beta1 and osteopontin and indirectly affects collagen mRNA expression in the human heart. Cardiovasc Res 46, 463-475.

Landomesser, U., Drexler, H., 2003. oxidative stress, the renin-angiotensin system, and atherosclerosis. european heart journal 5, A3-A7.

Lenz, T., Sealey, J.E., Maack, T., James, G.D., Heinrikson, R.L., Marion, D., Laragh, J.H., 1991. Half-life, hemodynamic, renal, and hormonal effects of prorenin in cynomolgus monkeys. Am J Physiol 260, R804-810.

Leung, P.S., Wong, T.P., Lam, S.Y., Chan, H.C., Wong, P.Y., 2000. Testicular hormonal regulation of the renin-angiotensin system in the rat epididymis. Life Sci 66, 1317-1324.

London, G.M., Pannier, B., Guerin, A.P., Marchais, S.J., Safar, M.E., Cuche, J.L., 1994. Cardiac hypertrophy, aortic compliance, peripheral resistance, and wave reflection in end-stage renal disease. Comparative effects of ACE inhibition and calcium channel blockade. Circulation 90, 2786-2796.

Macdougall, I.C., 1999. The role of ACE inhibitors and angiotensin II receptor blockers in the response to epoetin. Nephrol Dial Transplant 14, 1836-1841.

Matsumoto, N., Ishimitsu, T., Okamura, A., Seta, H., Takahashi, M., Matsuoka, H., 2006. Effects of imidapril on left ventricular mass in chronic hemodialysis patients. Hypertens Res 29, 253-260.

Methot, D., Silversides, D.W., Reudelhuber, T.L., 1999. In vivo enzymatic assay reveals catalytic activity of the human renin precursor in tissues. Circ Res 84, 1067-1072.

Mimran, A., Shaldon, S., Barjon, P., Mion, C., 1978. The effect of an angiotensin antagonist (saralasin) on arterial pressure and plasma aldosterone in hemodialysis-resistant hypertensive patients. Clin Nephrol 9, 63-67.

Morishita, Y., Hanawa, S., Chinda, J., Iimura, O., Tsunematsu, S., Kusano, E., 2011a. Effects of aliskiren on blood pressure and the predictive biomarkers for cardiovascular disease in hemodialysis-dependent chronic kidney disease patients with hypertension. Hypertens Res 34, 308-313.

Morishita, Y., Hanawa, S., Miki, T., Sugase, T., Sugaya, Y., Chinda, J., Iimura, O., Tsunematsu, S., Ishibashi, K., Kusano, E., 2011b. The association of plasma prorenin level with an oxidative stress marker, 8-OHdG, in nondiabetic hemodialysis patients. Clin Exp Nephrol 15, 398-404.

Nussberger, J., Wuerzner, G., Jensen, C., Brunner, H.R., 2002. Angiotensin II suppression in humans by the orally active renin inhibitor Aliskiren (SPP100): comparison with enalapril. Hypertension 39, E1-8.

Prescott, G., Silversides, D.W., Reudelhuber, T.L., 2002. Tissue activity of circulating prorenin. Am J Hypertens 15, 280-285.

Racki, S., Zaputovic, L., Mavric, Z., Vujicic, B., Dvornik, S., 2006. C-reactive protein is a strong predictor of mortality in hemodialysis patients. Ren Fail 28, 427-433.

Sadoshima, J., Izumo, S., 1993. Molecular characterization of angiotensin II--induced hypertrophy of cardiac myocytes and hyperplasia of cardiac fibroblasts. Critical role of the AT1 receptor subtype. Circ Res 73, 413-423.

Saracho, R., Martin-Malo, A., Martinez, I., Aljama, P., Montenegro, J., 1998. Evaluation of the Losartan in Hemodialysis (ELHE) Study. Kidney Int Suppl 68, S125-129.

Schaefer, R.M., Schaefer, L., Horl, W.H., 1994. Anaphylactoid reactions during hemodialysis. Clin Nephrol 42 Suppl 1, S44-47.

Shibasaki, Y., Masaki, H., Nishiue, T., Nishikawa, M., Matsubara, H., Iwasaka, T., 2002. Angiotensin II type 1 receptor antagonist, losartan, causes regression of left ventricular hypertrophy in end-stage renal disease. Nephron 90, 256-261.

Siragy, H.M., 2000. AT(1) and AT(2) receptors in the kidney: role in disease and treatment. Am J Kidney Dis 36, S4-9.

Suzuki, H., Kanno, Y., Sugahara, S., Ikeda, N., Shoda, J., Takenaka, T., Inoue, T., Araki, R., 2008. Effect of angiotensin receptor blockers on cardiovascular events in patients undergoing hemodialysis: an open-label randomized controlled trial. Am J Kidney Dis 52, 501-506.

Suzuki, H., Kanno, Y., Sugahara, S., Okada, H., Nakamoto, H., 2004. Effects of an angiotensin II receptor blocker, valsartan, on residual renal function in patients on CAPD. Am J Kidney Dis 43, 1056-1064.

Takahashi, A., Takase, H., Toriyama, T., Sugiura, T., Kurita, Y., Ueda, R., Dohi, Y., 2006. Candesartan, an angiotensin II type-1 receptor blocker, reduces cardiovascular events in patients on chronic haemodialysis--a randomized study. Nephrol Dial Transplant 21, 2507-2512.

Takemitsu, T., Ichihara, A., Kaneshiro, Y., Sakoda, M., Kurauchi-Mito, A., Narita, T., Kinouchi, K., Yamashita, N., Itoh, H., 2009. Association of (pro)renin receptor mRNA expression with angiotensin-converting enzyme mRNA expression in human artery. Am J Nephrol 30, 361-370.

Tarng, D.C., Huang, T.P., Wei, Y.H., Liu, T.Y., Chen, H.W., Wen Chen, T., Yang, W.C., 2000. 8-hydroxy-2'-deoxyguanosine of leukocyte DNA as a marker of oxidative stress in chronic hemodialysis patients. Am J Kidney Dis 36, 934-944.

Vaidyanathan, S., Bigler, H., Yeh, C., Bizot, M.N., Dieterich, H.A., Howard, D., Dole, W.P., 2007. Pharmacokinetics of the oral direct renin inhibitor aliskiren alone and in combination with irbesartan in renal impairment. Clin Pharmacokinet 46, 661-675.

van Ampting, J.M., Penne, E.L., Beek, F.J., Koomans, H.A., Boer, W.H., Beutler, J.J., 2003. Prevalence of atherosclerotic renal artery stenosis in patients starting dialysis. Nephrol Dial Transplant 18, 1147-1151.

Vlahakos, D.V., Hahalis, G., Vassilakos, P., Marathias, K.P., Geroulanos, S., 1997. Relationship between left ventricular hypertrophy and plasma renin activity in chronic hemodialysis patients. J Am Soc Nephrol 8, 1764-1770.

Wagner, J., Jan Danser, A.H., Derkx, F.H., de Jong, T.V., Paul, M., Mullins, J.J., Schalekamp, M.A., Ganten, D., 1996. Demonstration of renin mRNA, angiotensinogen mRNA, and angiotensin converting enzyme mRNA expression in the human eye: evidence for an intraocular renin-angiotensin system. Br J Ophthalmol 80, 159-163.

Wang, A.Y., Li, P.K., Lui, S.F., Sanderson, J.E., 2004. Angiotensin converting enzyme inhibition for cardiac hypertrophy in patients with end-stage renal disease: what is the evidence? Nephrology (Carlton) 9, 190-197.

Wauters, J.P., Waeber, B., Brunner, H.R., Guignard, J.P., Turini, G.A., Gavras, H., 1981. Uncontrollable hypertension in patients on hemodialysis: long-term treatment with captopril and salt subtraction. Clin Nephrol 16, 86-92.

Weidmann, P., Maxwell, M.H., Lupu, A.N., Lewin, A.J., Massry, S.G., 1971. Plasma renin activity and blood pressure in terminal renal failure. N Engl J Med 285, 757-762.

Zannad, F., Kessler, M., Lehert, P., Grunfeld, J.P., Thuilliez, C., Leizorovicz, A., Lechat, P., 2006. Prevention of cardiovascular events in end-stage renal disease: results of a randomized trial of fosinopril and implications for future studies. Kidney Int 70, 1318-1324.

Zheng, S., Nath, V., Coyne, D.W., 2007. ACE inhibitor-based, directly observed therapy for hypertension in hemodialysis patients. Am J Nephrol 27, 522-529.

Zoccali, C., Benedetto, F.A., Mallamaci, F., Tripepi, G., Fermo, I., Foca, A., Paroni, R., Malatino, L.S., 2000. Inflammation is associated with carotid atherosclerosis in dialysis patients. Creed Investigators. Cardiovascular Risk Extended Evaluation in Dialysis Patients. J Hypertens 18, 1207-1213.

8

Diagnosis and Treatment of Primary Aldosteronism

Ozlem Tiryaki* and Celalettin Usalan
Gaziantep University School of Medicine, Department of Nephrology
Turkey

1. Introduction

Primary aldosteronism (PAL) is a clinical disorder characterized by excessive production and release of aldosterone from the cortical zona glomerulosa of the adrenal gland. The high level of circulating aldosterone increases sodium reabsorption with potassium loss in the distal tubule, leading to mild hypernatremia, hypertension (HTN), severe hypokalemia, and alkalosis. [1,2] Primary aldosteronism, as originally described by Conn in the 1950s.[3,4] (PAL)is characterized by an increased secretion of aldosterone that seems to be autonomous of the renin–angiotensin system, as the secretion of renin is suppressed. PAL represents the most common form of secondary hypertension.[5,6] In recent years, the large- scale hypertension trials, It is now widely recognized that PAL is much more common than previously thought, being present in up to 5–13% of unselected hypertensive patients[7] and in resistant HTN (BP above goal with three or more antihypertensive medications) with a reported prevalence of 20% to 23% in this group of patients.[5,8] As older age and obesity are 2 of the strongest risk factors for uncontrolled hypertension, the incidence of resistant hypertension will likely increase as the population becomes more elderly and heavier. The prognosis of resistant hypertension is unknown, but cardiovascular risk is undoubtedly increased as patients often have a history of long-standing, severe hypertension complicated by multiple other cardiovascular risk factors such as obesity, sleep apnea, diabetes, and chronic kidney disease.[5] In ALLHAT, older age, higher baseline systolic blood pressure, LVH, and obesity all predicted treatment resistance as defined by needing 2 or more antihypertensive medications. Overall, the strongest predictor of treatment resistance was having CKD as defined by a serum creatinine of ≥1.5 mg/dL. Other predictors of the need for multiple medications included having diabetes mellitus and living in the southeastern United States. African-American participants had more treatment resistance, as did women, such that black women had the lowest control rate (59%) and non-black men the highest (70%).[8] Furthermore, experimental and clinical studies showed that excess aldosterone has detrimental effects on the heart, brain and kidneys that are partly hypertension-independent.[9] Patients diagnosed with PAL, compared with patients with essential hypertension seems to increase the left ventricular wall thickness.[10] In addition, aldosterone excess appears to independently increase the risk of cardiac fibrosis.[11] Likewise, mineralocorticoid receptor blockage has been showed to diminish the effects of aldosterone

* Corresponding Author

on PAI-1 levels. In recent years, clinical trials have demonstrated an additive effect of combined ACEI and aldosterone receptor antagonism on cardiovascular morbidity and mortality.[12,13] The mechanism, named aldosterone escape, referring to chronic ACEI that leads aldosterone to return to baseline concentrations, might clarify the additional effects of aldosterone on PAI-1 levels.[14,15] We study, administration of an ACEI (fosinopril) and an ACEI plus aldosterone antagonist (spironolactone) both caused a significant decrease in PAI-1 levels, which might be attributed to aldosterone escape.[16]

Several studies have shown that patients with either aldosterone-producing adenoma (APA) or idiopathic hyperaldosteronism (IHA) appear to have increased cardiovascular morbidity compared with age-, sex-, and systolic and diastolic BP-matched patients with essential hypertension.[17,18] Patients with PAL, stroke, MI and significantly increased risk of atrial fibrillation.[19] Optimal BP control and specific management of aldosterone excess by either adrenalectomy or medical treatment with mineralocorticoid receptor (MR) antagonists is fundamental for the prevention of cardiovascular events in patients with PA.[20]

The adverse effects of aldosterone excess stress the importance of establishing the diagnosis of PAL and its underlying cause. The most common subtypes of PAL are APA (35% of cases) and IHA (60% of cases).[21] Many other subtypes of PAL have also been described, including primary or unilateral adrenal hyperplasia (2%), pure aldosterone-secreting adrenocortical carcinoma (<1%) and ectopic aldosterone- secreting tumours (e.g. neoplasms in the ovary or kidney) (<0.1%).[22]

2. Clinical findings

2.1 Symptoms and signs

The most common findings in PAL, moderate or severe hypertension and hypokalemia. PAL patients are often resistant hypertension, hypertension in these patients usually need to take control of multiple drug use. In recent studies, only a minority of patients with PAL (9–37%) had hypokalemia.[23] Although hypokalemia is considered the hallmark of hyperaldosteronism, the majority of patients with PAL have normal serum potassium levels. Hypokalemia is believed to be a late manifestation of PAL and many patients with PAL may present with HTN well before they develop hypokalemia. [6,23] Most symptoms of PAL are attributed to hypokalemia, which include muscle weakness, cramping, transient paralysis, palpitations, headache, or polyuria.[22]

Half the patients with an APA and 17% of those with idiopathic hyperaldosteronism (IHA) had serum potassium concentrations less than 3.5 mmol/liter.[24] Thus, the presence of hypokalemia has low sensitivity and specificity and a low positive predictive value for the diagnosis of PAL. Separation of IHA and APA, IHA to be treated medically, surgically corrected if the APA is very important because of an illness.

2.2 Laboratory findings

The recently published Guidelines for diagnosis and treatment of PAL outlined for the first time the categoriesof hypertensive patients with relatively high prevalence of PAL who should undergo a screening test. [1] The screening test should be performed in all patients with: **1)** resistant hypertension; **2)** hypertension grade 2 or 3; **3)** hypertension and spontaneous or diuretic-induced hypokalaemia **4)** hypertension with adrenal incidentaloma; **5)**hypertension and a family history of early-onset hypertension or cerebrovascular accident at a young age (<40 year); **6)** all hypertensive first-degree relatives of patients with PAL.

There is a general consensus that aldosterone:renin ratio (ARR) is the most reliable available means for PAL screening; however there is no agreement on either the ARR cut-off or whether the absolute aldosterone level should also be taken into account. Aldosterone/renin ratios (ARRs) were calculated from these values using the following Formula (ARR): Plasma aldosterone (ng/dL)/Plasma renin (ng/mL-h) . Individuals with an ARR of ≥30 were suspected of having primary aldosteronism, while an ARR of <30 was considered normal.[1] However, it is now recognized the prevalence is higher (5-13% of all patients with hypertension) when the PAC to PRA ratio (ARR) is used to screen for PAL. Measurements of PAC and PRA are recommended for the diagnosis of PAL.

Several factors affect ARR, the most important being antihypertensive therapy: mineralocorticoid receptor antagonists and diuretics lead to false-negative results and thus should always be withdrawn for at least 4–6 weeks (6– 8 for spironolactone); dihydropyridine calcium channel blockers, angiotensin-converting enzyme inhibitors, angiotensin II receptor antagonists can potentially, but infrequently, led to false-negative results[25]; in contrast, beta-blockers and central 2-agonists can cause false positives.[26] The direct renin inhibitor aliskiren lowers PRA, resulting in false-positive ARR for renin measured as PRA and false negatives for renin measured.[1]

An increased ARR is not diagnostic by itself, and PAL must be confirmed by demonstrating over- production of aldosterone. The Endocrine Society guidelines recommend the following four confirmatory tests; an oral sodium test, saline infusion test, fludrocortisone test and captopril challenge test.[1] Patients should receive 12.8 g sodium chloride for 3 days in the oral sodium loading test. The captopril challenge test shows excellent sensitivity despite relatively low specificity and due to its simplicity can be performed at the outpatient clinic.

Oral sodium loading test: This test is performed to evaluate the suppression of aldosterone by oral sodium loading. The oral sodium loading test is also not practical in hypertensive patients because of their high-salt intake, and the intravenous saline infusion test is not common as it is dangerous for elderly patients or those with left ventricular hypertrophy or a previous myocardial infarction, all of which are commonly complicated by PAL. The most commonly used test to verify the diagnosis oarl sodium loading test. Patients should increase their sodium intake to 200 mmol/d (6 g/d) for 3 day, verified by 24-h urine sodium content. Patients should receive adequate slow-release potassium chloride supplementation to maintain plasma potassium in the normal range. Urinary aldosterone is measured in the 24-h urine collection from the morning of d 3 to the morning of day 4. PAL is unlikely if urinary aldosterone is lower than 10 μg/24 h (27.7 nmol/ d) in the absence of renal disease where PAL may coexist with lower measured urinary aldosterone levels. Elevated urinary aldosterone excretion >12 μg/24 h (>33.3 nmol/d) at the Mayo Clinic, >14 μg/24 h (38.8 nmol/d) at the makes PAL highly likely.

Urinary aldosterone levels greater than 12 mcg/24 hours indicate failure to suppress the aldosterone production by high salt intake and is diagnostic of PAL with over 90% sensitivity and specificity.[22]

Saline loading test: Patients stay in the recumbent position for at least 1 h before and during the infusion of 2 liters of 0.9% saline iv over 4 h, starting at 08:00–09:30 h. Blood samples for renin, aldosterone, cortisol, and plasma potassium are drawn at time zero and after 4 h, with blood pressure and heart rate monitored throughout the test. Post infusion plasma aldosterone < 5 ng/dl make the diagnosis of PAL unlikely, and levels >10 ng/ dl are a very probable sign of PAL. Values between 5 and 10 ng/dl are indeterminate.[34] SLT is contraindicated in patients with severe HTN, chronic kidney failure, HF, cardiac dysrhythmias, or severe hypokalemia.

Captopril challenge test: Patients receive 25–50 mg captopril orally after sitting or standing for at least 1 h. Blood samples are drawn for measurement of PRA, plasma aldosterone, and cortisol at time zero and at 1 or 2 h after challenge, with the patient remaining seated during this period. Plasma aldosterone is normally suppressed by captopril (>30%). The test is considered positive if SA remains greater than 12 ng/dL or ARR is greater than 26.[28] This test has a higher sensitivity (100% versus 95.4%) and specificity (67% to 91% versus 28.3%) over the baseline screening tests, and is easier to perform than the SLT.

Fludrocortisone suppression test: Fludrocortisone suppression is the standard test used to confirm the diagnosis of PAL. Fludrocortisone (Florinef) is given 0.1 mg every 6 hours orally together with high oral sodium of 200 mmol (6 g) per day for 4 days. Potassium supplement should be given to maintain a close to normal serum potassium level. Upright SA and PRA are obtained on day 4 of the test. SA greater than 6 ng/dL is indicative of failure to suppress the aldosterone production and is diagnostic of PAL; PRA should be suppressed to less than 1 ng/mL/hour. FST requires hospital admission because of hypokalemia associated with testing as well as the need for frequent blood samples to monitor serum potassium levels. This test is contraindicated in patients with severe HTN or heart failure (HF). [1,27]

3. Imaging studies

3.1 Adrenal computed tomography

Imaging of adrenal glands by computed tomography (CT) and magnetic resonance imaging (MRI) is frequently used to detect an adrenal mass in patients with positive screening and confirmation tests. [29]

APA may be visualized as small hypodense nodules (usually<2 cm in diameter) on CT. IHA adrenal glands may be normal on CT or show nodular changes. Aldosterone-producing adrenal carcinomas are almost always more than 4 cm in diameter, but occasionally smaller, and like most adrenocortical carcinomas have a suspicious imaging phenotype on CT. [30]

A high resolution CT scan with 2–3 mm cuts represents the best available technique for identifying adrenal nodules that can be an APA, primary unilateral adrenal hyperplasia or bilateral adrenal hyperplasia.[31] According to the Endocrine Society guidelines, MRI, CT or both should be performed in patients with primary aldosteronism to identify the rare but large aldosterone-producing carcinoma.[32] However, as MRI is more expensive and has a lower spatial resolution than CT, MRI has no advantage over CT in subtype evaluation of primary aldosteronism.[1]

Half of APAs are <20 mm in diameter and up to 42% are <6 mm in diameter, therefore, most patients with primary aldosteronism attributable to an APA who can be cured with surgery have a small or very small tumor.[33] Other surgically curable subtypes of primary aldosteronism, such as primary aldosteronism caused by primary unilateral adrenal hyperplasia or multinodular unilateral adrenocortical hyperplasia, have nodular lesions that are also most often very small (<10 mm in diameter), which makes them hardly detectable with CT or MRI. In addition, a nonfunctioning adrenal mass (incidentaloma) can also be present in a patient with primary aldosteronism either with a small APA or with unilateral adrenocortical hyperplasia, both of which are undetectable with CT. Moreover, in a patient with primary aldosteronism, an adrenal nodule can be an APA, a macronodule of hyperplasia attributable to idiopathic hyperaldosteronism,[34] or a macronodule attributable to primary unilateral adrenal hyperplasia.[35]

3.2 Adrenal venous sampling

There are an increasing number of reports that adenal vein sampling (AVS) is the gold standard test to differentiate unilateral from bilateral disease in patients with PAL. The Endocrine Society guidelines state that AVS is the "standard test to differentiate unilateral from bilateral causes of [primary aldosteronism]. [1] Adrenal venous sampling is a difficult procedure as the right adrenal vein is small, with the success rate depending on the proficiency of the angiographer. AVS is expensive, technically demanding and carries a tiny, but not negligible, risk of adrenal-vein rupture.[36]

In a study where AVS was used as the gold standard for diagnosis, CT scans mistakenly suggested that one-quarter of patients had an APA; correctly identified a unilateral or bilateral excess of aldosterone only in half of all patients; falsely suggested a bilateral adrenal hyperplasia in one-fifth of patients with a unilateral source of aldosterone excess; and in some patients identified an APA in the wrong adrenal gland.[34]

Rapid cortisol assays during AVS to monitor cortisol levels can reduce the failure rate of AVS. We have developed a new rapid cortisol assay using immunochromatography, in which cortisol concentrations can be measured within 6 min. (briefly explain false positive rates etc., in this method- should this be used in conjunction with CT?) Using this technique, the success rate of AVS has improved to 93% .[37]

4. Treatment

At our institution, we support the recommendation from the Endocrine Society guidelines[1] that a lateralized aldosterone secretion should be demonstrated before undertaking surgery in patients who are candidates for general anesthesia and wish to achieve long-term cure. The goal of treatment for PAL is focused on the normalization of circulating aldosterone or aldosterone receptor blockade to prevent the morbidity and mortality associated with HTN, hypokalemia and end-organ damage.[29] Management strategies should take patient characteristics and desires into consideration. Surgical treatment may not be appropriate for all patients with unilateral hypersecreting adrenal mass but may be reasonable for those with bilateral hypersecretion.

4.1 Medical treatment

Medical management with a mineralocorticoid receptor (MR) antagonist is recommended for patients who do not undergo surgery. Medical treatment is recommended for patients with bilateral hypersecreting adrenal lesions or for those with unilateral lesion who are not optimal for or who do not want surgical treatment (see Pharmacotherapy for hyperaldosteronism). Medications that block aldosterone action are effective for the treatment of hypokalemia and HTN and these include nonselective (spironolactone) and selective aldosterone receptor antagonists (eplerenone). Amiloride is not an aldosterone receptor antagonist and is not effective in controlling HTN in PAL but may be used for its potassium sparing property.

Prior studies on the efficacy of spironolactone in treating resistant HTN have used 25 to 50 mg daily dosing, whereas true PAL may require larger daily doses up to 100 to 400 mg. The onset of action on BP may be slow. Measurements of PRA are not necessary but may be an indication that an optimal dose of the medication has been prescribed when it is no longer suppressed.

Spironolactone is a nonselective MR antagonist with significant antiandrogenic and progestational activities responsible for its most common side effects (gynecomastia, erectile dysfunction and abnormal menstrual cycles) [2]. Eplerenone is a selective MR antagonist without antiandrogen or progesterone agonist activity: it has 60% of the potency of spironolactone in vivo and should be administered twice daily given its short half-life. Combined therapy with a small dose of spironolactone and amiloride may alleviate these undesirable consequences.[29] Eplerenone, a more selective mineralocorticoid receptor blocker, also effectively reduces BP in patients with resistant hypertension Eplerenone has a beter adverse reaction profile because it has substantially less binding affinity to androgen and progesterone receptors than spironolactone.

4.2 Surgical treatment

Laparoscopic adrenalectomy is currently the best treatment, and can be performed during a short hospital stay at a very low operative risk.[38-39] This surgery has cured primary aldosteronism in 33–72% of patients and resulted in marked improvements in 40–50% of patients.[40,41] Approximately one-third of all PAL patients has clear lateralization of aldosterone production and will benefit from unilateral adrenalectomy. Laparoscopic adrenectomy is the most suitable therapy for APA or unilateral adrenal hyperplasia. After adrenalectomy hypertension is cured in around 50% of patients with APA (range 33–70%) [3] with the remaining patients showing a significant reductions in blood pressure and number of antihypertensive drugs. Chronic suppression of the renin-angiotensin axis may cause transient postoperative hypoaldosteronism and a liberal sodium diet should be allowed to prevent hyperkalemia after the surgery. An I.V. infusion of 0.9% sodium chloride every 8 to 12 hours may be necessary to avoid postoperative intravascular volume depletion. All antihypertensive medications, especially spironolactone and amiloride, should be withheld and other BP medications may be cautiously reinstituted as needed within a few days. The data on follow-up assessment of the remaining adrenal gland after surgery is scanty. Postoperative SA, PRA, and ARR are commonly repeated.[17] These authors also periodically obtained CT scan in their patients at 1 to 3 yearly intervals because they have observed that the remaining adrenal gland could slowly increase in size, become nodular or develop adenoma after surgery.

Of note, adrenalectomy in APA patients has also been reported to improve self-assessed quality of life. [42] A recent study suggests that, for reasons which are incompletely understood, unilateral adrenalectomy may be beneficial in carefully selected patients with bilateral PA. [43]

5. Conclusion

Until recently, aldosterone excess was thought to play a minor role in the development of hypertension. Beginning in the early 1990s, however, reports from investigators worldwide have found that primary aldosteronism is common in patients with hypertension, with prevalence rates of 10 to 15%. In patients with severe or resistant hypertension, the prevalence of primary aldosteronism is even higher, with a prevalence of approximately 20%. Approximately 30% to 60% of APA patients are improved or have resolution of HTN and hypokalemia with normal SA and PRA after unilateral adrenectomy. HTN is normally resolved within 1 to 6 months and patients with persistent HTN are more likely to be older, require more than two antihypertensive drugs preoperatively, or have a longer duration of HTN or underlying renal dysfunction. The postoperative BP in those with persistent HTN is usually easier to control with fewer medications. The cardiovascular complications of patients who achieve optimal BP control with or without medications eventually decrease to the levels of those with essential HTN. Partial reversal of renal dysfunction, regression of LVM and improved diastolic left ventricular function have been demonstrated after successful treatment of PAL. It has been reported that adrenalectomy for APA is more cost-effective than long-term medical therapy.

6. References

[1] Funder JW, Carey RM, Fardella C, Gomez-Sanchez CE, Mantero F, Stowasser M, . Case detection, diagnosis, and treatment of patients with primary aldosteronism: An endocrine society clinical practice guideline. *J Clin Endocrinol Metab* 2008;93(9):3266-3281.

[2] Stowasser M, Gordon RD, Rutherford JC, Nikwan NZ, Daunt N, Slater GJ. Diagnosis and management of primary aldosteronism. *J Renin Angiotensin Aldosterone Syst.* 2001;2(3):156-169.

[3] Conn, J. W. in *Hypertension: Pathophysiology and Treatment* 768–780 (McGraw-Hill, New York, 1977).

[4] Conn, J. W. A concluding response. *Arch. Intern. Med.* 1969; 123: 154–155 .

[5] Calhoun DA, Jones D, Textor S, et al. Resistant hypertension: diagnosis, evaluation, and treatment: a scientifi c statement from the american heart association professional education committee of the Council for High Blood Pressure Research. *Circulation.* 2008;117(25):e510-e526.

[6] Mosso L, Carvajal C, González A, et al. Primary aldosteronism and hypertensive disease. *Hypertension.* 2003;42(2):161-165.

[7] Rossi, G. P. *et al.* A prospective study of the prevalence of primary aldosteronism in 1,125 hypertensive patients. *J. Am. Coll. Cardiol.* 2006;48: 2293–2300 .

[8] Cushman WC, Ford CE, Cutler JA, et al. Success and predictors of blood pressure control in diverse North American settings: the antihypertensive and lipid-lowering treatment to prevent heart attack trial (ALLHAT). J Clin Hypertens (Greenwich). 2002;4:393-404.

[9] Rocha R, Stier Jr CT. Pathophysiological effects of aldosterone inncardiovascular tissues. Trends Endocrinol Metab. 2001;12:308–14.

[10] Tsioufis C, Tsiachris D, Dimitriadis K, Stougiannos P, Missovoulos P, Kakkavas A, et al. Myocardial and aortic stiffening in the early course of primary aldosteronism. Clin Cardiol. 2008;31:431–6.

[11] Brilla CG, Weber KT. Reactive and reparative myocardial fibrosis in arterial hypertension in the rat. Cardiovasc Res. 1992;26:671–7.

[12] Pitt B, Zannad F, Remme WJ, Cody R, Castaigne A. The effect of spironolactone on morbidity and mortality in patients with severe heart failure. *N. Engl. J. Med.* 1999; 341: 709–17.

[13] Williams ES, Miller JM. Results from late-breaking clinical trial sessions at the American College of Cardiology 51st Annual Scientific Session. *J. Am. Coll. Cardiol.* 2002; 40: 1–18.

[14] Brown NJ, Agırbasli MA, Williams GH, Litchfield WR, Vaughan DE. Effect of activation and inhibition of the rennin angiotensin system on plasma PAI-1 in humans. *Hypertension* 1998; 32: 965–71.

[15] Struthers AD. Aldosterone escape during ACE inhibitor therapy in chronic heart failure. *Eur. Heart J.* 1995; 16: 103–6.,

[16] Tiryaki O, Usalan C, Buyukhatipoglu H. Effect of combined angiotensin-converting enzyme and aldosterone inhibition on plasma plasminogen activator inhibitor type 1 levels in chronic hypertensive patients. Nephrology (Carlton), 2010;15(2): 211-5.

[17] Rossi, G. P., Pessina, A. C. And Heagerty, A. M. Primary aldosteronism: an update on screening, diagnosis and treatment. *J. Hypertens.* 2008;26, 613–621.

[18] Born-Frontsberg E, Reincke M, Rump LC, Hahner S, Diederich S, Lorenz R, et al. Cardiovascular and cerebrovascular comorbidities of hypokalemic and normokalemic primary aldosteronism: results of the German Conn's Registry. J Clin Endocrinol Metab. 2009;94:1125–30.

[19] Milliez P, Girerd X, Plouin PF, Blacher J, Safar ME, Mourad JJ. Evidence for an increased rate of cardiovascular events in patients with primary aldosteronism. J Am Coll Cardiol. 2005;45:1243–8.

[20] Catena C, Colussi G, Nadalini E, Chiuch A, Baroselli S, Lapenna R, et al. Cardiovascular outcomes in patients with primary aldosteronism after treatment. Arch Intern Med. 2008;168:80–5.

[21] Davis WW, Newsome Jr HH, Wright Jr LD, Hammond WG, Easton J, Bartter FC. Bilateral adrenal hyperplasia as a cause of primary aldosteronism with hypertension, hypokalemia and suppressed renin activity. Am J Med. 1967;42:642–7.

[22] Young WF. Primary aldosteronism: renaissance of a syndrome. Clin Endocrinol (Oxf). 2007;66:607–18.

[23] Mulatero P, Stowasser M, Loh KC, et al. Increased diagnosis of primaryaldosteronism, including surgically correctable forms, in centers from fi ve continents. *J Clin Endocrinol Metab.* 2004;89(3):1045-1050.

[24] Kaplan NM. Is there an unrecognized epidemic of primary aldosteronism? Pro. *Hypertension.* 2007;50(3):447-453.

[25] Stowasser M, Gordon RD, Rutheford JC, et al. Diagnosis and management of primary aldosteronism. J Renin Angiotensin Aldosterone Syst. 2001;2:156–69.

[26] Mulatero P, Rabbia F, Milan A, et al. Drug effects on aldosterone/plasma renin activity ratio in primary aldosteronism. *Hypertension.* 2002;40(6): 897-902.

[27] Mulatero P, Milan A, Fallo F, et al. Comparison of confirmatory tests for the diagnosis of primary aldosteronism. *J Clin Endocrinol Metab.* 2006;91(7):2618-2623.

[28] Castro OL, Yu X, Kem DC. Diagnostic value of the post-captopril test in primary aldosteronism. *Hypertension.* 2002;39(4):935-938.

[29] Young WF Jr. Minireview: Primary Aldosteronism—changing concepts in diagnosis and treatment. *Endocrinology.* 2003;144(6):2208-2213.

[30] Young Jr WF. Clinical practice. The incidentally discovered adrenal mass. N Engl J Med 2007;356:601–610

[31] Mulatero P, Bertello C, Verhovez A, et al. Differential diagnosis of primary aldosteronism subtypes. Curr Hypertens Rep. 2009;11:217–23.

[32] Rossi, G. P., Vendraminelli, R., Cesari, M. and Pessina, A. C. A thoracic mass with hypertension and hypokalaemia. *Lancet* 2000; 356, 1570.

[33] Omura, M., Sasano, H., Fujiwara, T., Yamaguchi, K. & Nishikawa, T. Unique cases of unilateral hyperaldosteronemia due to multiple adrenocortical micronodules, which can only be detected by selective adrenal venous sampling. *Metabolism* 2002;51, 350–355.

[34] Magill SB, Raff H, Shaker JL, et al. Comparison of adrenal vein samplingand computed tomography in the differentiation of primary aldosteronism. *J Clin Endocrinol Metab.* 2001;86(3):1066-1071

[35] Goh, B. K. *et al.* Primary hyperaldosteronism secondary to unilateral adrenal hyperplasia: an unusual cause of surgically correctable hypertension. A review of 30 cases. *World J. Surg.2007;*31, 72–79.

[36] Daunt, N. Adrenal vein sampling: how to make it quick, easy, and successful. *Radiographics* 2005; 25 (Suppl. 1), S143–S158.

[37] Takeda Y, Yoneda T, Karashima S, Demura M, Hashimoto A, Mori S, et al. Rapid assay of cortisol during adrenal vein sampling is useful for the diagnosis of primary aldosteronism. J Hypertens. 2009;27 Suppl 4:S446.

[38] Jeschke, K. *et al.* Laparoscopic partial adrenalectomy in patients with aldosterone-producing adenomas: indications, technique, and results. *Urology* 2003;61, 69–72.

[39] Meria, P., Kempf, B. F., Hermieu, J. F., Plouin, P. F. & Duclos, J. M. Laparoscopic management of primary hyperaldosteronism: clinical experience with 212 cases. *J. Urol.* 2003;169, 32–35.

[40] Sawka, A. M. *et al.* Primary aldosteronism: factors associated with normalization of blood pressure after surgery. *Ann. Intern. Med.* 2001;135, 258–261.

[41] Lumachi, F. *et al.* Long-term results of adrenalectomy in patients with aldosterone-producing adenomas: multivariate analysis of factors affecting unresolved hypertension and review of the literature. *Am. Surg.*2005; 71, 864–869.

[42] Sukor N, Kogovsek C, Gordon RD, et al. Improved quality of life, blood pressure, and biochemical status following laparoscopic adrenalectomy for unilateral primary aldosteronism. J Clin Endocrinol Metab. 2010;95:1360–4.

[43] Sukor N, Gordon RD, Ku YK, et al. Role of unilateral adrenalectomy in bilateral primary aldosteronism: a 22-year single center experience. J Clin Endocrinol Metab. 2009;94:2437–45.